Case Presentations in Medical Ophthalmology

Case Presentations in Medical Ophthalmology

Jack J. Kanski MD, MS, FRCS
Consultant Ophthalmologist

Teifi E. James MRCP, FRCS
Senior House Officer

Prince Charles Eye Unit, King Edward VII Hospital, Windsor

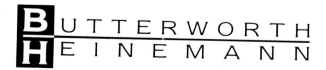

● PART OF REED INTERNATIONAL P.L.C.

OXFORD LONDON GUILDFORD BOSTON
MUNICH NEW DELHI SINGAPORE SYDNEY
TOKYO TORONTO WELLINGTON

First published 1991

© **Butterworth–Heinemann Ltd, 1991**

British Library Cataloguing in Publication Data

Kanski, Jack J.
  Case presentations in medical ophthalmology.
  1. Ophthalmology
  I. Title   II. James, Teifi E.
  617.7

  ISBN 0 7506 1184 7

Library of Congress Cataloging in Publication Data

Kanski, Jack J.
   Case presentations in medical ophthalmology / Jack J. Kanski and
Teifi E. James
     p.   cm.
   Includes index.
   ISBN 0–7506–1184–7 :
   1. Ophthalmology—Case studies.   I. James, Teifi E.   II. Title.
   [DNLM: 1. Eye Diseases—case studies.   2. Eye Diseases—
   examination questions.   WW 18 K16x]
   RE69.K36   1991
   617.7—dc20
   DNLM/DLC   90—15123

Printed in Scotland by Cambus Litho Ltd, Glasgow
Bound by Hartnolls Ltd, Bodmin, Cornwall

Preface

Apart from being the *sine qua non* of higher professional training in general medicine and its subspecialities, the Membership of the Royal College of Physicians (or equivalent) is desired by doctors wishing to pursue careers in other fields. As candidates continue to attempt the examination, many of them well prepared, the examiners are having to diversify the questions, especially the slide section, to include photographs of conditions that most candidates will not immediately recognize. Although this has beneficial implications for the overall standards of medicine, it also results in increasing problems with preparation for the examination.

This book presents a selection of short case histories each followed by three questions to help focus the reader's thoughts. In cases where the diagnosis is not immediately apparent, the questions can act as a pointer to the type of answer desired by the examiners. Although this book is primarily aimed at physicians preparing for higher examinations, we are sure that it will also be of value to ophthalmologists in training and to medical students.

We are very grateful to Miss Daphne Bannister for taking many of the photographs.

J.J.K.
T.E.J.
Windsor, 1990

Contents

Introduction

Examination of the eyes as part of a general physical examination is very important. Most 'self-respecting' diseases have ocular manifestations or associations which should be within the diagnostic domain of the physician. One must be aware of these eye conditions, be able to examine the eyes proficiently and stylishly, and be able to arrive at a sound differential diagnosis for three reasons:

- To know when to refer to an ophthalmologist.
- To aid general medical diagnosis.
- To pass the MRCP examination or equivalent.

Your examination should begin as you approach the patient. Observation and awareness are crucial to your success. For example, amputees may be diabetic, patients in wheelchairs can have multiple sclerosis and those with grossly diminished acuity or diplopia could have problems with the mandatory handshake. It has been said that a polite introduction and a good farewell to the patient give you two marks out of five for a short case. Irrespective of whether or not this is actually true, a respectful and affable approach will certainly gain favour with the examiners. Passing membership is a bit like passing a driving test, it is not enough to be capable, you have to demonstrate to the examiners that you are performing safely, carefully and 'be seen to be checking your rearview mirror' or its medical equivalent. The five important steps in the examination of a short case are:

- Politely introduce yourself.
- Request the patient's permission to examine.
- Perform a stylish, thorough and swift examination.
- Thank the patient.
- Present your findings and diagnosis in a coherent, confident and well-organized fashion.

Examination Techniques

When taken to a patient, the examiner will tell you what to do. Clues as to the required extent of your examination should be gleaned from the way the command is phrased. In examining the eyes, there are a limited number of options. The first is 'at a glance' diagnosis such as 'What do you notice about Mr Jones' eyes?'. The second is more specific instructions such as: 'Examine Mrs Smith's vision', 'Examine this patient's pupils', 'Does this patient have a visual field defect?', 'Examine this patient's eye movements' or 'Look at this man's fundi'. Each of these possibilities will now be discussed.

'At a glance' diagnosis

If asked 'What do you notice about Mr Jones' eyes?' do not embark on a full examination of the extraocular movements and fundi. First look at the face as a whole – Does it look normal? Is there asymmetry? – then inspect the eyes. If no obvious diagnosis leaps at you, be systematic and think of the following, possible, 'at a glance' diagnoses:

- Eyelids – ptosis, ectropion, entropion, heliotrope rash, periorbital oedema etc.
- Eyes – proptosis, glass eye, subconjunctival haemorrhage, cataract, arcus senilis etc.

Visual acuity

It is important to ensure that the patient is wearing the appropriate spectacles.

Very rough assessment

Introduce yourself, proffer a hand and say 'Please look at my eyes – can you see them?' – if the patient cannot see your eyes, then visual acuity is probably less than 6/60; if the patient can see your eyes, then check each eye separately by alternately occluding the patient's eyes with the back of your hand.

Detailed assessment

Ideally, measure visual acuity with a Snellen chart at 6 metres. If a Snellen chart is not available, ask the patient to read a newspaper. Roughly speaking the ability to read newsprint indicates a visual acuity of at least 6/12.

If visual acuity is less than 6/60 (i.e. the patient cannot see the top letter of the test type) proceed as follows:

- Hold up three fingers about half a metre in front of the patient and ask 'How many fingers do you see?' (Figure 1). If the response is correct, visual acuity is recorded as 'counting fingers (CF) at half metre' and the test is terminated. If the patient cannot see your fingers, even when they are very close, proceed as follows.
- Move your hand up and down close to the patient's eye and ask him if he can see it moving. If he can, visual acuity is recorded as 'hand movements (HM)'. If the patient cannot see HM, proceed as follows.
- Shine a pen torch on and off into his eye and ask 'Tell me when you see the light'; according to the response visual acuity is then recorded as either 'no light perception (no PL)' or 'light perception (PL)'.

Common errors

Common errors to avoid are:

- Failure to test each eye separately.
- Failure to ensure that the patient is wearing the appropriate spectacles when testing visual acuity (i.e. not reading spectacles when testing distance vision!).

Causes of poor visual acuity

In order of frequency these are:

- Uncorrected refractive error – by far the most common cause.
- Organic eye disease – e.g. corneal opacities, cataract, diabetic retinopathy, macular degeneration.
- Amblyopia – most frequently due to a childhood squint.
- Neurological lesions of the visual pathways.

The pupils

The pupils should be round and regular. They should also react to light and constrict to a near target as part of the near response which

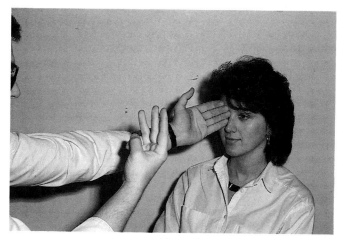

Figure 1

consists of (1) convergence of the two visual axes, (2) accommodation of the lenses so that the target is in focus and (3) constriction of the pupils.

Size and symmetry

- Ask the patient to view a distant object such as a picture on a wall.
- Direct a dim light onto the face from below so that both pupils are seen simultaneously.
- Assess their size and symmetry – ideally the size should be measured with a millimetre rule.

Note: important points

- About 20% of normal subjects have pupils of slightly different size (physiological anisocoria) which is of no significance.
- In physiological anisocoria, the difference in pupil size is the same irrespective of the extent of illumination.
- In pathological anisocoria, the difference in pupil size is dependent on the degree of illumination.
- A unilateral visual deficit does not affect pupillary size.

Light reflex

- Ask the patient to view a distant object to avoid pupillary constriction on looking at the torch as part of the near response.
- Bring the beam from lateral to medial so that the beam falls onto the right pupil and observe the reactions of both pupils.
- Repeat for the left eye.

If the afferent arc is intact, the direct reaction should equal the consensual reaction.

Note: the swinging flashlight test is used to detect an afferent pupillary defect (Marcus Gunn pupil) as follows:

- Shine the light onto the right eye and then move rapidly from one eye to the other and back again.

The reactions of the pupils are interpreted as follows:

- In normal eyes both pupils will remain constricted.
- In the presence of a Marcus Gunn pupil (as in retrobulbar neuritis or central retinal artery occlusion), the pupil on the affected side dilates on direct light stimulation and constricts on consensual stimulation. Thus, in the presence of a right Marcus Gunn pupil, the swinging flashlight test will result in both pupils dilating as the light falls on the right eye and both pupils constricting when the left is stimulated.

Near reflex

- Ask the patient to slightly elevate his chin and view a distant object.
- Ask the patient to look at his fingertip about 2 inches (5 cm) in front of his nose.
- Grade the degree of constriction ($+1$ to $+4$).

Note: you must know the causes of large and small pupils and of one large and one small pupil (anisocoria) etc.

Eye movements

The actions of the extraocular muscles must be assessed in the six cardinal positions of gaze as follows (Figure 2):

- Ask the patient to look at the tip of your index finger (or some other target such as a white hat pin) and to follow the finger as it is moved.
- If you suspect an ophthalmoplegia (nerve palsy), ask the patient if he or she has double vision (bearing in mind that the patient has to see with both eyes to experience diplopia) and then find in which position of gaze the diplopia is worse (i.e. there is maximal separation of the two images) and where it may be abolished. This should permit you to decide which muscles are affected. Saccadic eye movements are tested by asking the patient to look rapidly from side to side (use your hands as targets) and up and down. Nystagmus should be sought and you should know the different types and their significance (i.e. horizontal, vertical, see-saw and nystagmoid movements associated with internuclear ophthalmoplegia).

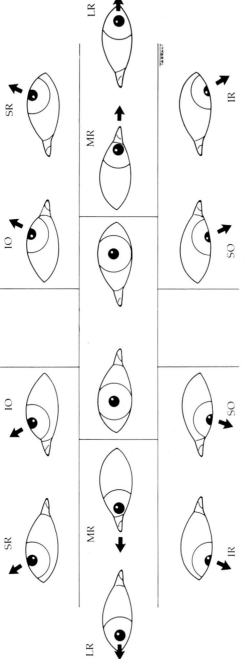

Figure 2 SR = superior rectus; IR = inferior rectus; MR = medial rectus; LR = lateral rectus; IO = inferior oblique; SO = superior oblique

Visual fields

Confrontational tests are used to detect hemianopias and altitudinal visual field defects. Essentially, when performing confrontation tests the examiner compares the patient's visual field with his own while in a face-to-face position about half a metre from the patient. The main confrontation tests are: finger-counting, simultaneous finger-counting, colour comparison and confrontation using a hat pin.

Finger-counting

This is performed as follows:

- Sit about half a metre in front of the patient.
- Ask the patient to cover his left eye with his left hand.
- Ask the patient to look directly with his right eye at your left eye.
- Present one finger, two fingers, five fingers or a clenched fist (but not three or four fingers) in the patient's left upper visual quadrant and ask the patient 'How many fingers do you see?' (Figure 3a).
- Repeat for the remaining three quadrants and then for the other eye.

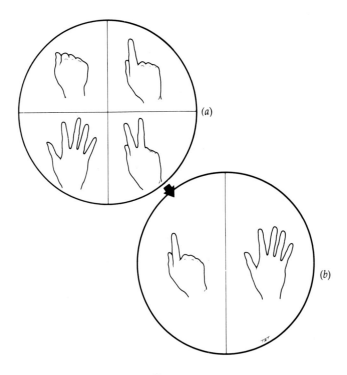

Figure 3

Simultaneous finger-counting

This is performed if the finger-counting test is normal. Its purpose is to detect the phenomenon of 'extinction' in which the defective hemifield appears intact when tested alone, but when tested with simultaneous stimuli a subtle defect may become apparent. The test is performed by asking the patient to count the number of fingers presented simultaneously by both of the examiner's hands in the two hemifields (Figure 3b).

Colour comparison

This is a useful screening test for early temporal visual field defects caused by chiasmal compression. It is performed as follows:

- Present the patient with two fairly large red objects such as hat pins or drop bottle tops about 2 inches (5 cm) to either side of fixation.
- Ask the patient 'Is there any difference in the colour of the two objects?'.

In a patient with an early temporal visual field defect, the colour of the object held in the nasal field will appear more red than the one held in the temporal field.

Confrontation using a hat pin

This is performed as follows:

- Start by holding the hat pin behind the patient's head (Figure 4).
- Slowly bring the pin forward in an arc until it is perceived.
- Repeat for the other three quadrants and then for the other eye.

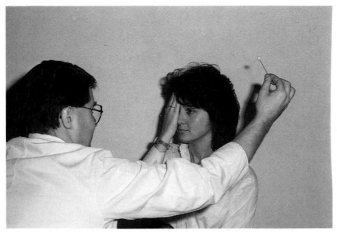

Figure 4

Ophthalmoscopy

This technique can be mastered only by practice and cannot be learned from a book. Try to spend at least one half-day in your local eye department looking at fundi. Remember the following points:

- The pupils can be dilated quickly and safely by using tropicamide 1% drops (Mydriacyl) – there is no need to counteract with pilocarpine.
- First examine the red reflex by looking at the patient's pupils through the ophthalmoscope from about an arm's length away (Figure 5).

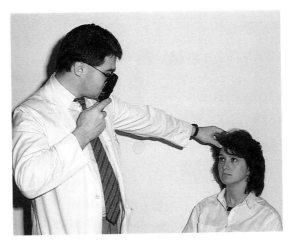

Figure 5

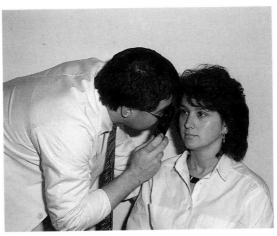

Figure 6

- The most common cause of an abnormal red reflex is cataract. Other causes are an opacity in the cornea and blood in the vitreous.
- Use your right eye when examining the patient's right eye and vice versa (Figure 6).
- It is easier to examine a highly myopic eye while looking through the patient's spectacles.

Case Presentations and Questions

Case 1

This 50-year-old man complains of blurring of vision in his right eye. When the photograph was taken he was closing both eyes (Figure 1a).

Questions

1. What are the signs and diagnosis?
2. What could be the cause of his blurred vision?
3. Is referral to an ophthalmologist appropriate?

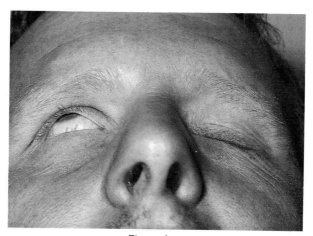

Figure 1a

Case 2

While shaving one morning, this 25-year-old man noticed that his left pupil was larger than the right (Figure 2a).

Questions

1. What are the signs?
2. What is the differential diagnosis?
3. What pharmacological tests may be helpful?

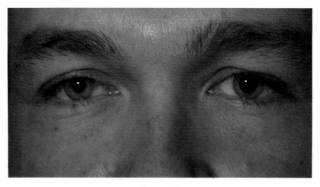

Figure 2a

Case 3

Two days ago this 75-year-old woman developed sudden and severe frontal headache and drooping of her right upper eyelid (Figure 3a).

Questions

1. What are the signs and probable diagnosis?
2. What is the possible aetiology?
3. What investigations would you order?

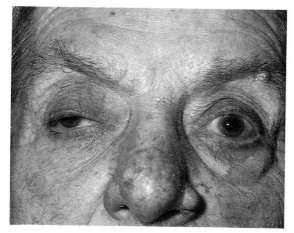

Figure 3a

Case 4

This 42-year-old man developed insulin-dependent diabetes 7 months ago. On waking yesterday he noticed double vision. The photograph was taken when he was looking to his left (Figure 4a).

Questions

1. What are the signs and diagnosis?
2. What type of diplopia will he have?
3. Is he likely to have diabetic retinopathy?

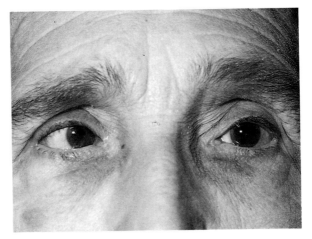

Figure 4a

Case 5

Four months ago this 40-year-old woman developed gradually pro-gressive vertical diplopia. When the photograph was taken she was looking up (Figure 5a).

Questions

1. What are the signs and probable diagnosis?
2. What associated systemic signs may be present?
3. What medical conditions may cause vertical diplopia?

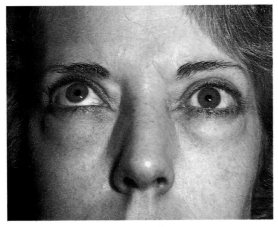

Figure 5a

Case 6

Nine months ago this 45-year-old woman developed intermittent drooping of her eyelids (Figure 6a).

Questions

1. What is the differential diagnosis?
2. What special investigations may be helpful?
3. Is referral to an ophthalmologist appropriate?

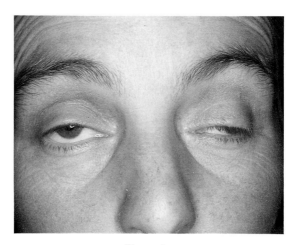

Figure 6a

Case 7

This 50-year-old patient with severe Graves' disease complains of constant ocular irritation (Figure 7a).

Questions

1. Why do patients with Graves' disease have lid retraction?
2. What are other medical causes of lid retraction?
3. What could be the cause of the patient's ocular discomfort?

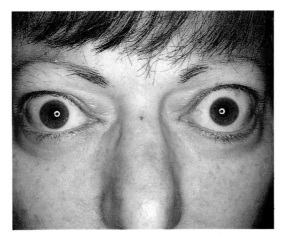

Figure 7a

Case 8

This 65-year-old man has had bilateral ocular discomfort for several months. Three weeks ago he developed a gradual greying of vision in his left eye which has increased during the last few days (Figure 8a).

Questions

1. What are the signs and probable diagnosis?
2. What could be the cause of his visual symptoms?
3. What are the therapeutic options?

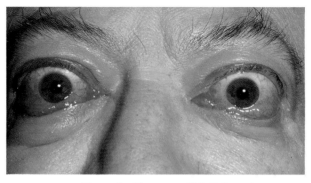

Figure 8a (Courtesy of Mr P. Rosen)

Case 9

Three days ago this 75-year-old woman developed a sudden rushing noise in her head and pain and redness of her right eye (Figure 9a).

Questions

1. What are the signs and probable diagnosis?
2. What other clinical signs may be present?
3. What is the management?

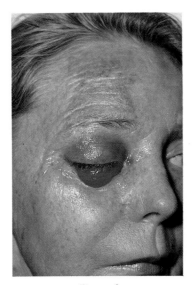

Figure 9a

Case 10

One year ago this 38-year-old man developed a painless and gradually increasing proptosis of his left eye (Figure 10a).

Questions

1. Which systemic diseases (excluding thyroid) may cause proptosis?
2. What are the most common non-systemic causes of proptosis?
3. What special investigations are indicated?

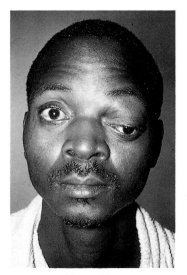

Figure 10a

Case 11

This 20-year-old woman has had very poor vision in her left eye for several years (Figure 11a).

Questions

1. What are the signs and systemic diagnosis?
3. What could be the cause of her visual impairment?
4. What other systemic problems could she have?

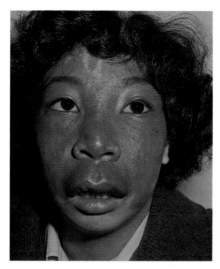

Figure 11a

Case 12

This 75-year-old man has had a blind right eye since the age of 5 (Figure 12a).

Questions

1. What are the signs and systemic diagnosis?
2. How is this disorder classified?
3. What could be the cause of the blindness in his right eye?

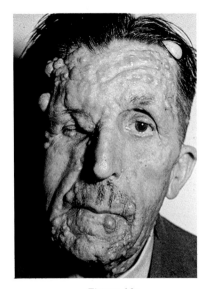

Figure 12a

Case 13

This young man has epilepsy and is mentally handicapped (Figure 13a).

Questions

1. What are the signs and diagnosis?
2. What are the ocular manifestations?
3. What central nervous system lesions could he have?

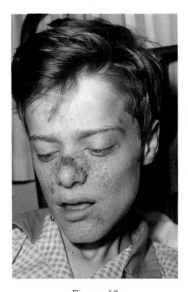

Figure 13a

Case 14

Ten days ago this 51-year-old woman developed a rash and now has a
red and sore right eye (Figure 14a).

Questions

1. What are the signs and diagnosis?
2. What may be the cause of her red eye?
3. Is referral to an ophthalmologist appropriate?

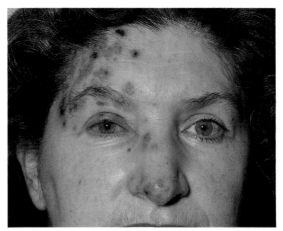

Figure 14a

Case 15

Two weeks ago this 36-year-old man developed fever and arthralgia. Three days ago he developed bilateral conjunctivitis and a skin rash (Figure 15a).

Questions

1. What are the signs and probable systemic diagnosis?
2. What could be the aetiology?
3. What is the visual prognosis?

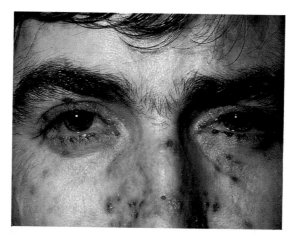

Figure 15a

Case 16

Four days ago this 25-year-old man developed a bilateral ocular discharge. In the morning his eyelids are stuck together and he has to bathe them open (Figure 16a).

Questions

1. What are the signs and diagnosis?
2. What are the possible systemic associations?
3. What is the visual prognosis?

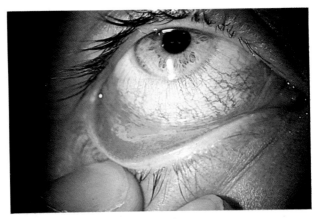

Figure 16a

Case 17

This 56-year-old woman developed chronic ocular irritation in both eyes 6 months ago. This photograph was taken following instillation of a dye into the inferior fornix (Figure 17a).

Questions

1. What are the signs and diagnosis?
2. What are the possible systemic associations?
3. What is the treatment?

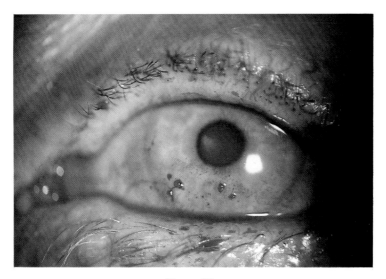

Figure 17a

Case 18

This 35-year-old man developed acute photophobia and redness in his left eye 2 days ago. This photograph was taken after the instillation of a mydriatic (Figure 18a).

Questions

1. What are the signs and diagnosis?
2. What are the possible systemic associations?
3. What is the treatment?

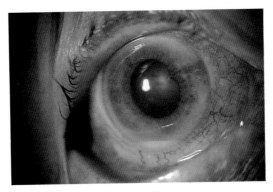

Figure 18a

Case 19

This 20-year-old man has been treated with steroid drops to both eyes on and off for 8 years. Four months ago he noticed very blurred vision in his left eye (Figure 19a).

Questions

1. What are the signs and diagnosis?
2. What are the possible systemic associations?
3. What are the ocular complications of long-term steroid drops?

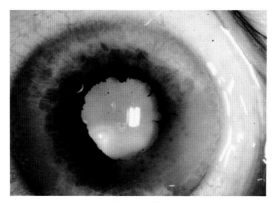

Figure 19a

Case 20

This 68-year-old woman developed severe pain, watering and blurring of vision in her left eye 3 weeks ago (Figure 20a).

Questions

1. What are the signs and diagnosis?
2. What are the possible systemic associations?
3. Why is this patient's eyesight at risk?

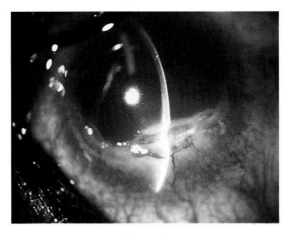

Figure 20a

Case 21

This is the eye of a 60-year-old man who has no visual symptoms. The other eye has an identical appearance (Figure 21a).

Questions

1. What are the signs and diagnosis?
2. What systemic conditions could he have?
3. What is the likelihood of the patient having a retinopathy?

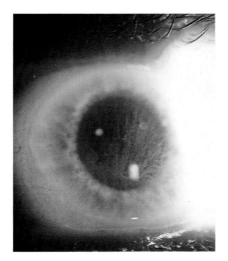

Figure 21a

Case 22

This is the asymptomatic eye of a 56-year-old woman with long-standing polyarthritis (Figure 22a).

Questions

1. What are the signs and diagnosis?
2. What non-articular systemic complications could the patient have?
3. What other eye complications could she develop?

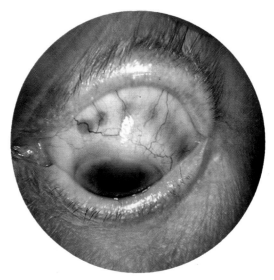

Figure 22a

Case 23

This is the red reflex of the left eye of a 30-year-old man (Figure 23a).

Questions

1. What are the signs and the probable systemic disease?
2. Name two other systemic diseases which may have similar ocular abnormalities.
3. What other ocular complications could this patient have?

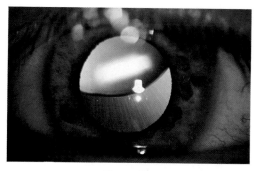

Figure 23a

Case 24

This is the red reflex of a 45-year-old man who has noticed a gradual deterioration of vision in both eyes (Figure 24a).

Questions

1. What is the diagnosis?
2. What are the possible systemic associations?
3. What is the treatment?

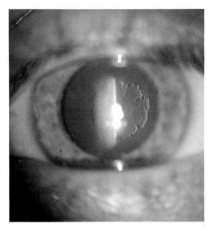

Figure 24a

Case 25

This 35-year-old woman developed a painless loss of vision in her left eye one week ago. On examination she had a left Marcus Gunn pupil and defective colour vision (Figure 25a).

Questions

1. What are the signs and probable diagnosis?
2. What systemic problems may she have?
3. What other ocular complications could she subsequently develop?

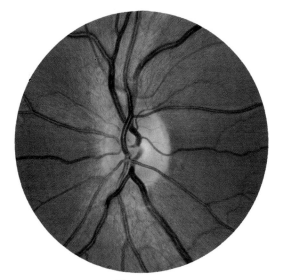

Figure 25a

Case 26

Nine months ago this 52-year-old woman developed mild headaches and a gradual loss of vision in her right eye. On examination visual acuity was extremely poor and there was a right Marcus Gunn pupil (Figure 26a).

Questions

1. What is the diagnosis?
2. What are the possible causes?
3. What special investigations may be appropriate?

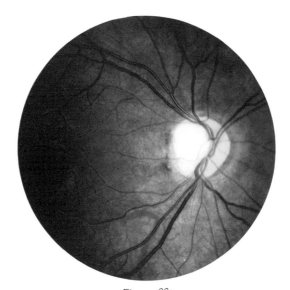

Figure 26a

Case 27

This 30-year-old woman complains of headaches but has no visual symptoms (Figure 27a). The other eye has a similar appearance.

Questions

1. What are the signs and probable diagnosis?
2. What are the possible causes?
3. What condition could give rise to a similar appearance?

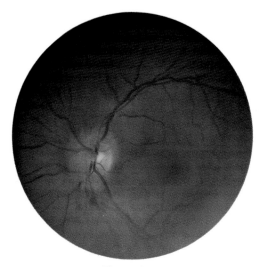

Figure 27a

Case 28

Two days ago this 75-year-old man noted a sudden loss of vision in his right eye (Figure 28a). On examination visual acuity was very poor and there was a marked Marcus Gunn pupil.

Questions

1. What are the signs and probable diagnosis?
2. What special investigations would be appropriate?
3. What is the treatment?

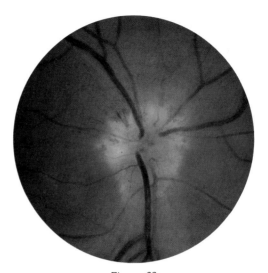

Figure 28a

Case 29

During the last 2 weeks this 66-year-old man has noticed three transient attacks of loss of vision in his right eye lasting between 5 and 10 minutes (Figure 29a).

Questions

1. What are the signs and probable diagnosis?
2. What systemic problems could the patient develop?
3. What special investigations would you consider?

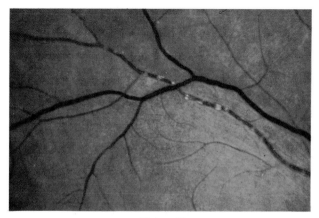

Figure 29a

Case 30

One hour ago this 60-year-old woman noticed a sudden painless loss of vision in her left eye (Figure 30a). On examination visual acuity was extremely poor and there was a Marcus Gunn pupil.

Questions

1. What are the signs and diagnosis?
2. What treatment would you carry out?
3. What are the possible systemic associations?

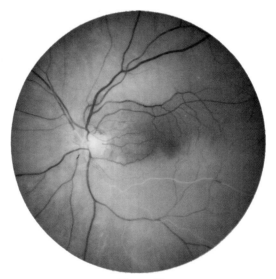

Figure 30a

Case 31

This is the fundus of a 30-year-old patient with renal failure due to chronic nephritis (Figure 31a).

Questions

1. What are the signs and diagnosis?
2. How could the ocular lesions progress?
3. What other ocular complications could the patient develop?

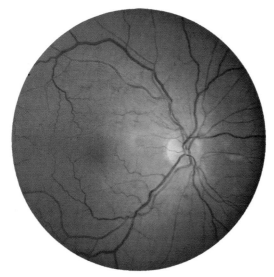

Figure 31a

Case 32

Two days ago this 68-year-old man developed severe loss of vision in his left eye (Figure 32a).

Questions

1. What are the signs and diagnosis?
2. What are the possible systemic associations?
3. What is his visual prognosis?

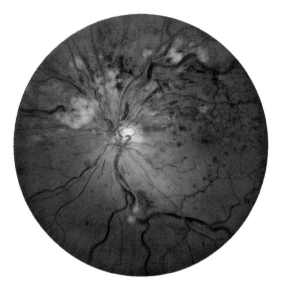

Figure 32a

Case 33

This 55-year-old woman was told by her optician that she had diabetes and was advised to see her GP (Figure 33a). However, all tests for diabetes were negative. The other eye had a similar appearance.

Questions

1. What are the signs and diagnosis?
2. Is referral to an ophthalmologist appropriate?
3. What is her visual prognosis?

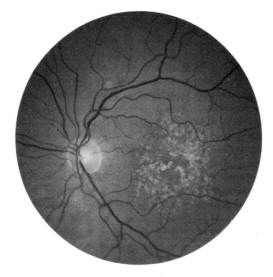

Figure 33a

Case 34

This is the eye of a 60-year-old, non-insulin-dependent diabetic with normal visual acuity (Figure 34a). The fundus in the other eye is normal.

Questions

1. What are the signs and diagnosis?
2. Is referral to an ophthalmologist appropriate?
3. What is the earliest clinical sign of diabetic retinopathy?

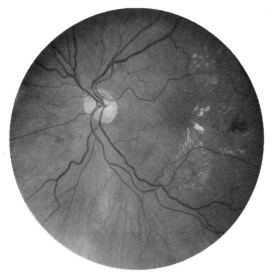

Figure 34a

Case 35

This 65-year-old diabetic complains of difficulty reading the share prices in the *Financial Times* despite recently obtaining new reading spectacles from his optician (Figure 35a).

Questions

1. What is the diagnosis?
2. Is referral to an ophthalmologist appropriate?
3. What special investigations may the ophthalmologist perform?

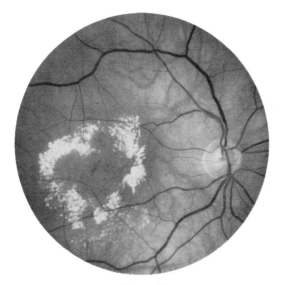

Figure 35a

Case 36

This 45-year-old diabetic was found to have abnormal fundi at a routine visit to the diabetic clinic (Figure 36a).

Questions

1. What are the signs?
2. Is referral to an ophthalmologist appropriate?
3. What systemic factors may worsen diabetic retinopathy?

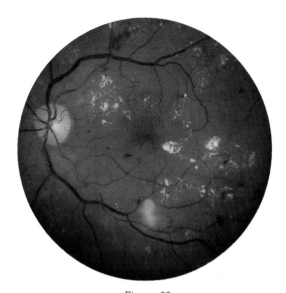

Figure 36a

Case 37

This is the fundus of a 35-year-old, insulin-dependent diabetic who has no visual symptoms (Figure 37a).

Questions

1. What are the signs?
2. Is referral to an ophthalmologist appropriate?
3. Apart from retinopathy what other eye complications may diabetic patients develop?

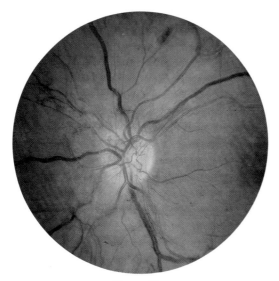

Figure 37a

Case 38

This patient is undergoing laser treatment for diabetic retinopathy (Figure 38a).

Questions

1. What are the principles of laser photocoagulation?
2. What are the main indications for laser therapy in diabetic patients?
3. Are there any potential complications of laser therapy?

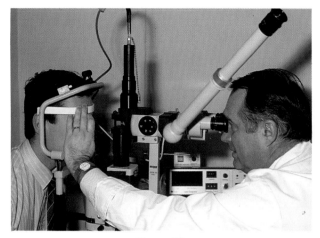

Figure 38a

Case 39

This man has had several laser treatments for proliferative diabetic retinopathy to his right eye. This morning he suddenly developed many thousands of tiny floaters followed by severe blurring of vision in the same eye (Figure 39a). His left eye has been completely blind for 2 years.

Questions

1. What are the signs and diagnosis?
2. What is the management?
3. What could be the cause of blindness in his left eye?

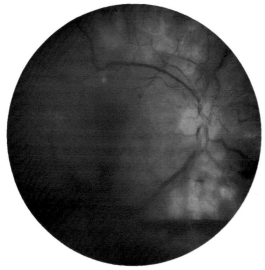

Figure 39a

Case 40

Three weeks ago this 35-year-old man developed floaters and blurred vision in his left eye (Figure 40a).

Questions

1. What are the signs and diagnosis?
2. What are the possible systemic associations?
3. What other ocular complications could the patient develop?

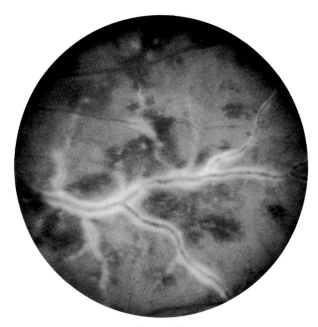

Figure 40a

Case 41

Two weeks ago this 22-year-old man noticed slight blurring of vision and floaters in his right eye (Figure 41a). Three years ago he had similar symptoms and was treated with tablets.

Questions

1. What are the signs and diagnosis?
2. What is the most common cause of this condition in the UK?
3. What are other possible systemic associations?

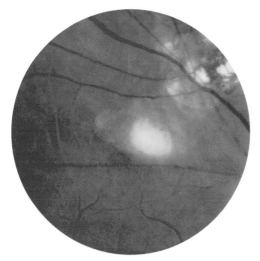

Figure 41a

Case 42

This 26-year-old man has been ill for over a year. Three months ago he developed a skin rash and 2 weeks ago he noticed blurred vision in both eyes (Figure 42a).

Questions

1. What are the signs and diagnosis?
2. What is the most common systemic association?
3. How are the ocular lesions treated?

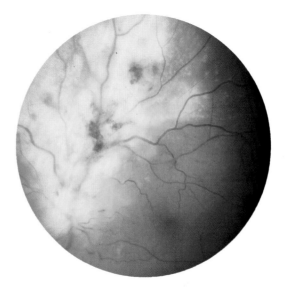

Figure 42a

Case 43

Two months ago this 45-year-old man noticed distortion of vision in his right eye (Figure 43a). Today his vision became much worse.

Questions

1. What are the signs and diagnosis?
2. What could be the cause of his recent visual loss?
3. What are the possible systemic associations?

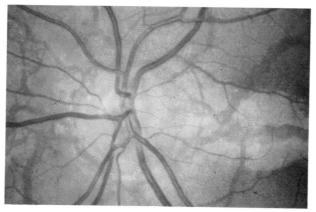

Figure 43a (Courtesy of Professor A. C. Bird)

Case 44

This is the fundus of a 16-year-old, mentally handicapped boy (Figure 44a).

Questions

1. What are the signs and diagnosis?
2. What visual symptoms could he have?
3. What are the possible systemic associations?

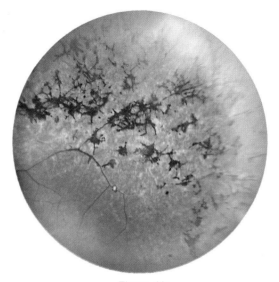

Figure 44a

Case 45

This 25-year-old woman was found to have an abnormal fundus by an optician (Figure 45a). Her brother is blind in both eyes and has ataxia.

Questions

1. What are the signs and diagnosis?
2. Why is her sight threatened?
3. What may be the cause of her brother's ataxia?

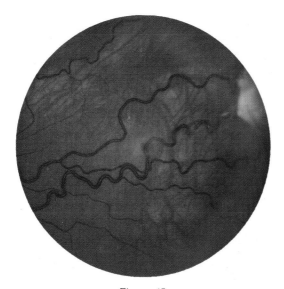

Figure 45a

Case 46

Five years ago this 55-year-old woman had a mastectomy for breast carcinoma. Two weeks ago she noticed slight blurring and distortion of vision of her left eye (Figure 46a).

Questions

1. What are the signs and diagnosis?
2. What is the differential diagnosis?
3. What other ocular problems could the patient develop?

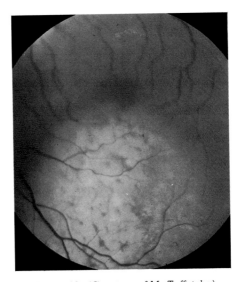

Figure 46a (Courtesy of Mr T. ffytche)

Case 47

This is the fundus of a 32-year-old man with carcinoma of the colon (Figure 47a).

Questions

1. What are the signs and diagnosis?
2. Why has he developed carcinoma at such an early age?
3. What other bowel disorders may be associated with ocular complications?

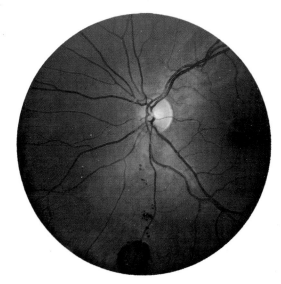

Figure 47a

Case 48

This chronic schizophrenic has been treated with drugs for many years. Recently he has complained of poor vision in both eyes (Figure 48a).

Questions

1. What are the signs?
2. What drug has been used to treat his schizophrenia?
3. What other systemically used drugs may be toxic to the retina or optic nerve?

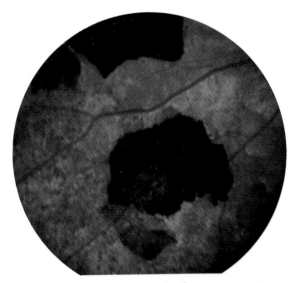

Figure 48a (Courtesy of Professor A. C. Bird)

Case 49

This is the blood film of a 10-year-old girl who developed a red eye 3 days ago (Figure 49a).

Questions

1. What does the blood film show?
2. What may be the cause of her red eye?
3. What other ocular complications could she develop?

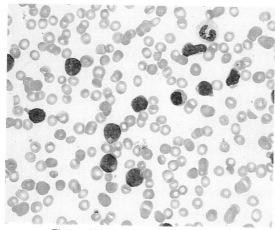

Figure 49a (Courtesy of Dr P. Mackie)

Case 50

This is the blood film of a 62-year-old man who complains of gradual visual impairment and difficulty in distinguishing colours (Figure 50a).

Questions

1. What does the blood film show?
2. What may be the cause of his visual symptoms?
3. What other ocular problems could he have?

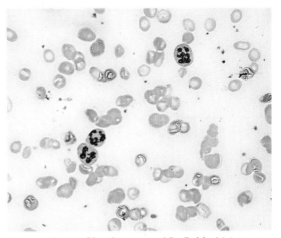

Figure 50a (Courtesy of Dr P. Mackie)

Answers and Discussions

Case 1

1. The signs are: inability to close the right eye and a positive Bell's phenomenon (rolling up of eye on attempting eyelid closure). The diagnosis is a *right facial nerve palsy*.
2. The probable cause of the blurred vision is *exposure keratopathy* due to drying of the cornea, particularly the lower half, because of inadequate spread of tears by the eyelids.

Note: the presence of exposure keratopathy increases the risk of secondary bacterial infection (bacterial keratitis) which is a very serious condition.

3. *Ophthalmic referral is advisable* because the early changes of exposure keratopathy are very subtle and can be detected only by

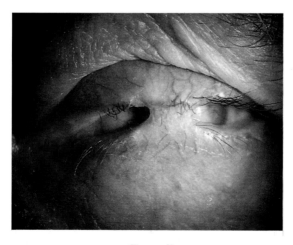

Figure 1b

examining the eye on a special microscope (slit lamp). The ophthalmologist will also advise on the most appropriate treatment:

- Mild or temporary cases are treated with artificial tear substitutes
  (hypromellose drops) and ointment (Lacri-lube) four or five times
  during the day and strapping the eyelids together at night.
- Severe or permanent cases may require a tarsorrhaphy in which
  the upper and lower lids are sutured together. Figure 1b shows a
  tarsorrhaphy in an eye with severe corneal scarring.

Case 2

1. The signs are: the left pupil is larger than the right (anisocoria), and
   both pupils are round and regular. Because the lower borders of
   both upper eyelids are nearly level with the pupillary margins the

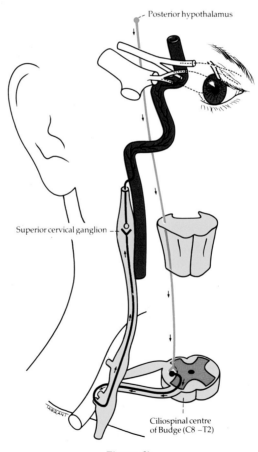

Posterior hypothalamus

Superior cervical ganglion

Ciliospinal centre
of Budge (C8 –T2)

Figure 2b

right lid must be lower than the left – this is suggestive of a mild right ptosis.

2. Differential diagnosis:
   - *Right Horner's syndrome* (oculosympathetic palsy) – causes include: Pancoast's tumour, malignant cervical lymph nodes, neck surgery, carotid and aortic aneurysms, cluster headaches, brain stem disease and congenital. Some cases are idiopathic. Figure 2b shows the anatomy of the sympathetic nerve supply to the eye.
   - *Left Holmes–Adie (tonic) pupil* – it is possible that the slight ptosis is incidental and the left pupil is abnormal (test for associated areflexia).
   - *Left pharmacological mydriasis* due to accidental instillation of drops.
3. Pharmacological tests:
   - In Horner's syndrome – *adrenaline 1:1000* drops will dilate a *post*ganglionic Horner's pupil but neither a *pre*ganglionic Horner's nor a normal pupil.
   - In Holmes–Adie pupil – *pilocarpine 0.1%* or *mecholyl 2.5%* drops will constrict the tonic pupil but not the normal pupil.

   Note: both are examples of denervation hypersensitivity – Horner's syndrome is sympathetic tone loss and Holmes–Adie pupil is parasympathetic tone loss.
   - In pharmacological mydriasis – *pilocarpine 1%* drops will constrict the normal, but not the large, pupil.

Case 3

1. The signs are: a moderate right ptosis and a right divergent strabismus. The diagnosis is an *acute right oculomotor (third) nerve palsy.*

   Figure 3b shows defective depression of the right eye due to paralysis of the inferior rectus muscle (the superior oblique muscle cannot depress the eye when it is in abduction).
2. The main causes of a painful third nerve palsy in this age group are:
   - *Posterior communicating aneurysm.*
   - *Diabetes* which may also cause a painless third nerve palsy.
   - *Giant cell arteritis.*
   - *Herpes zoster.*

   Note: 'medical' versus 'surgical' third nerve palsy.
   - Surgical lesions (e.g. aneurysms, tumours) typically compress the pial blood vessels which supply the superficially located parasympathetic pupillary nerve fibres and cause a dilated pupil.
   - Medical lesions (e.g. diabetes, hypertension) cause an ischaemic microangiopathy involving the vasa nervorum and cause infarction of the main trunk of the third nerve with sparing of the pupillary fibres.

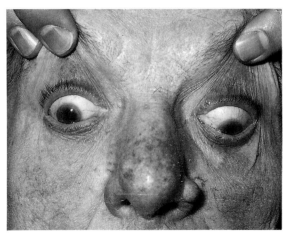

Figure 3b

3. Investigations
   - *Medical*: blood pressure, urinalysis and ESR.
   - *Cerebral arteriography* if an aneurysm is suspected.
   - *CT scan* in patients with associated cavernous signs.

   Note: The presence of diabetes or hypertension does not exclude an aneurysm.

Case 4

1. The signs are: failure of abduction of the left eye. The diagnosis is an *acute left abducens (sixth) nerve palsy*. Vascular ocular palsies in diabetics may occur suddenly. In the majority of cases spontaneous recovery usually occurs within a few months.

   Other important causes of an isolated sixth nerve palsy are:
   - Other vascular lesions such as hypertension.
   - Raised intracranial pressure associated with posterior fossa tumours or benign intracranial hypertension due to stretching of the sixth nerves over the petrous tip (a false-localizing sign).
   - Fractures of the base of the skull.
   - Acoustic neuromas which may damage the sixth nerve at the pontomedullary junction (remember to test corneal sensation).

   Note:
   - In contrast to third nerve palsy, aneurysms rarely cause a sixth nerve palsy.
   - About 25% of all isolated third, fourth and sixth nerve palsies are idiopathic and half of these recover spontaneously.
   - Myasthenia gravis can cause almost any type of ocular motility defect.

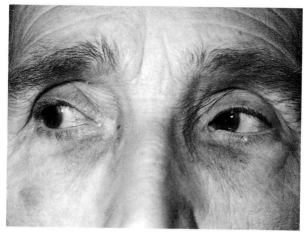

Figure 4b

2. *The diplopia will be horizontal* (worse on left gaze and least on right gaze). Figure 4b shows normal adduction of the left eye and no diplopia when the patient is looking to the right.
3. He will *not* have diabetic retinopathy because diabetic patients do not develop retinopathy until they have had diabetes for at least 5 years.

Case 5

1. The signs are: restriction of elevation of the left eye and bilateral infraorbital oedema. The probable diagnosis *is restrictive thyroid myopathy* involving the left inferior rectus muscle in which the fibrotic muscle fails to relax when the patient looks up.
   Note: in order of frequency, muscle involvement in thyroid ophthalmopathy is:
   • Inferior rectus which will restrict elevation.
   • Medial rectus which will restrict abduction.
   • Superior rectus which will restrict depression.
   • Lateral rectus which will restrict adduction.
2. Patients with thyroid ophthalmopathy may be *hyperthyroid, euthyroid* or *hypothyroid* (post-treatment). The classic triad of Graves' disease consists of: ophthalmopathy, clubbing of finger nails (acropathy) and pretibial myxoedema.
   Note:
   • In Graves' disease the eye signs are symmetrical (Figure 5b, right).

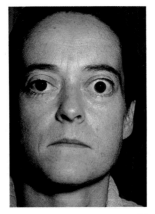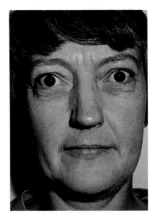

Figure 5b

- When ophthalmopathy occurs in isolation (ophthalmic Graves' disease) the eye signs are asymmetrical (Figure 5b, left).
- Ophthalmopathy does not occur with other causes of thyrotoxicosis (e.g. toxic nodular goitre).
3. Other causes of vertical diplopia are:
    - *Myasthenia gravis* typically causing intermittent vertical diplopia, although any or all of the extraocular muscles may be affected.
    - *Trochlear (fourth) nerve palsy* causing vertical diplopia which is worse on looking down (e.g. when eating).

Case 6

1. Differential diagnosis:
    - *Myasthenia gravis* is the most likely cause in this patient because she also has a left divergent squint. In myasthenia, the ptosis may be unilateral or bilateral and is typically worse following fatigue.
    - *Dystrophia myotonica* usually presents with myotonic features, ptosis and cataract. The extraocular muscles are unaffected.
    - *Ocular myopathy* is characterized by progressive bilateral ptosis and external ophthalmoplegia unassociated with diplopia. Some patients also have a pigmentary retinopathy and heart block (Kearns–Sayre syndrome).
    - *Involutional ptosis* is unassociated with any systemic disease.
2. Investigations:
    - Myasthenia gravis – *Tensilon test, antibodies* to anti-acetylcholine receptors and striated muscle and *chest X-ray, CT scan* or *MRI of anterior mediastinum* for thymic enlargement or thymoma.
    - Dystrophia myotonica is a *clinical diagnosis* – systemic features

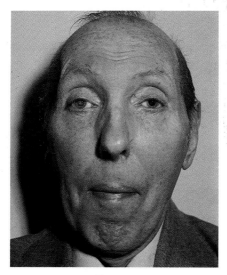

Figure 6b

include: myotonic facies, difficulties in releasing grip, muscle wasting, slurred speech, hypogonadism, cardiac anomalies and frontal baldness in men. Figure 6b shows a patient with myotonia and a right cataract.

- Ocular myopathy – *muscle biopsy* in some patients may show mitochondrial myopathy (inherited through the mother's cytoplasm).

3. Ophthalmic referral is advisable because some patients with severe non-myasthenic ptosis may require surgery.

Case 7

1. Lid retraction may be caused by a combination of:
   - *Overstimulation* of the sympathetically innervated *(Müller's) muscle* in the upper eyelids.
   - *Overaction of levator muscle* secondary to restrictive myopathy of the inferior rectus muscle.
   - *Restrictive myopathy and contraction* of the *levator* muscle itself.

   Note:
   - In many patients there is a combination of true lid retraction and pseudo-retraction due to associated proptosis.
   - Other lid signs in Graves' disease are: lid-lag (von Graefe's sign), staring appearance (Kocher's sign), infrequent blinking, fine tremor on lid closure and jerky movements on lid opening.

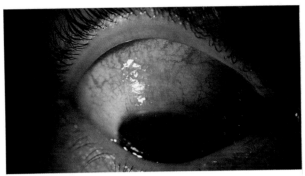

Figure 7b

2. Non-endocrine causes of lid retraction are:
   - *Aberrant regeneration of the third nerve* – this usually follows an acute traumatic or aneurysmal, but not a vascular, third nerve palsy.
   - *Overaction of the levator* associated with a *contralateral ptosis.*
   - *Collier's sign* of the dorsal mid-brain (Parinaud's syndrome).
   - *Familial periodic paralysis.*
3. The patient's symptoms may be due to:
   - *Exposure keratopathy* due to infrequent blinking – treat with lubricants (see Case 1).
   - *Superior limbic keratoconjunctivitis* which is much less common (Figure 7b). Refer to an ophthalmologist because management may be difficult.

Case 8

1. The signs are: bilateral lid retraction, proptosis, periorbital oedema and severe chemosis with the conjunctiva protruding over the margins of the lower eyelids. The most probable diagnosis is severe *thyroid ophthalmopathy.*
2. The most likely cause of his visual symptoms is *dysthyroid optic neuropathy* – a potentially blinding condition. It is thought to be caused by pressure on the optic nerve associated with apical orbital crowding by enlarged extraocular muscles. A CT scan shows enlarged extraocular muscles in thyroid ophthalmopathy (Figure 8b).

   Note: the main clinical features of dysthyroid optic neuropathy are:
   - Gradual greying of vision or colour desaturation.
   - Relative afferent pupillary conduction defect (Marcus Gunn pupil).
   - Variable visual field defects in 60% of cases.

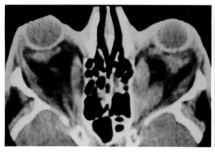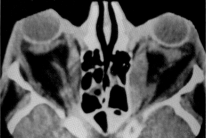

Figure 8b

- Fundus may show disc hyperaemia, optic atrophy or choroidal folds at the posterior pole. However, in many cases the fundus is normal.
3. Dysthyroid optic neuropathy requires prompt treatment:
   - *Systemic steroids* – initially 80–100 mg/day and then tapered over 3 months is usually the initial therapy. They may also reduce chemosis, proptosis and pain if used during the early course of the disease.
   - *Radiotherapy* – where steroid therapy is inappropriate.
   - *Orbital decompression* – if other measures fail or are inappropriate.

Case 9

1. The signs are: a complete right ptosis and severe chemosis. The most probable diagnosis is a *right carotid–cavernous fistula*. In this age group, the most likely cause is a spontaneous rupture of an intracavernous aneurysm or an atherosclerotic internal carotid artery. Postmenopausal hypertensive women are at particular risk. A fracture of the base of the skull may also cause a carotid–cavernous fistula.
2. Depending on severity the signs are:
   - *Pulsating proptosis* associated with a bruit over the right eye which may be abolished by ipsilateral carotid compression.
   - *Engorged blood vessels* on the surface of the eye (Figure 9b).
   - *Ophthalmoplegia* (particularly sixth nerve palsy) – common.
   - *Fundus changes* – vascular engorgement and central retinal vein occlusion.
   - *Raised intraocular pressure* (glaucoma) and *anterior segment ischaemia.*
3. The majority of carotid–cavernous fistulae are not life threatening and the eye is the major organ at risk. In many cases the fistula

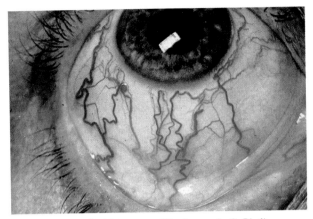

Figure 9b (Courtesy of Professor A. C. Bird)

closes spontaneously secondary to thrombosis of the cavernous sinus or its tributaries. The main indications for treatment are:

- Serious vision-threatening complications (e.g. glaucoma, exposure keratopathy).
- Persistent diplopia.
- Intolerable bruit or headache.

The many methods of treatment include *intravascular balloons* and *embolization* with glue or particulate matter.

Case 10

1. Systemic non-endocrine causes of proptosis include:
   - *Wegener's granulomatosis* – frequently involves the orbit by direct spread from diseased paranasal sinuses. Involvement is usually bilateral and associated with pain, chemosis and ophthalmoplegia.
   - *Lymphomas* – may involve any part of one or both orbits; Figure 10b shows bilateral, asymmetrical, lymphomatous, orbital involvement.
   - *Metastatic disease* – in adults the most common primary sites are bronchus, breast, prostate, kidney and gastrointestinal tract.
   - *Hand–Schüller–Christian disease* and *eosinophilic granuloma* – in children.
   - *Neurofibromatosis* – may cause proptosis by:
     - spheno-orbital encephalocele in infants, characterized by a pulsatile proptosis which is not associated with a bruit;
     - optic nerve glioma which typically develops between the ages of 4 and 8 years;
     - plexiform neuroma in the orbit.

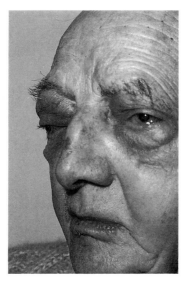

Figure 10b

2. Non-systemic causes of proptosis include:
   - *Carotid–cavernous fistula* (see Case 9).
   - *Inflammatory lesions*: orbital cellulitis, abscess and 'pseudo-tumour'.
   - *Primary orbital tumours*: haemangioma, lacrimal gland tumours, optic nerve sheath meningioma and rhabdomyosarcoma.
   - *Cystic lesions*: dermoid cysts and mucoceles.
3. Special investigations in patients with unexplained non-thyroid proptosis include: *plain X-rays*, *CT*, *MRI*, *ultrasonography* and *biopsy*.

Case 11

1. The signs are: a very large bilateral facial haemangioma with associated hypertrophy of the involved area of the face. The diagnosis is *Sturge–Weber syndrome* (encephalotrigeminal angiomatosis) which is the only phacomatosis that is not hereditary. The facial angioma (naevus flammeus) is present at birth and roughly involves the area of distribution of the first and second divisions of the trigeminal nerve. It is bilateral in about 10% of patients. The angioma may be associated with hypertrophy of the involved area of the face and occasionally it also involves the upper trunk and upper arms.

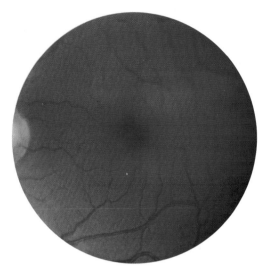

Figure 11b (Courtesy of Dr P. H. Morse)

2. Vision-threatening complications are:
   - *Developmental glaucoma* – in 30% of patients. It corresponds to the side of the facial angioma and is more common when the upper eyelid is involved.
   - *Diffuse ipsilateral angioma of the choroid* – in 40% of patients. The angioma gives the fundus a deep-red colour (Figure 11b).
   - *Angiomas* of the episclera, iris and ciliary body may also occur.
3. An associated ipsilateral angioma of the meninges and brain most frequently involving the parieto-occipital region may cause:
   - *Jacksonian-type epilepsy.*
   - *Hemiparesis and hemianopia.*
   - *Mental handicap* due to atrophy of the neighbouring cerebral cortex.

Case 12

1. The signs are: multiple facial cutaneous nodules and right facial hemiatrophy. The diagnosis is von Recklinghausen's *neurofibromatosis*. The facial lesions consist of cutaneous plexiform neuromas as well as the flabby and pedunculated fibromata mollusca.
2. The three main types of neurofibromatosis are:
   - *Neurofibromatosis 1* (peripheral form) – the most common.
   - *Neurofibromatosis 2* (central type) – mainly consists of bilateral acoustic neuromas with few if any cutaneous findings.
   - *Segmental type* – peripheral features are confined to one body segment.

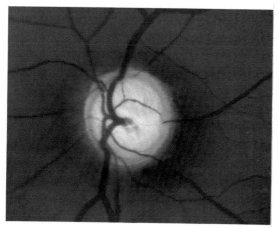

Figure 12b

3. The two main causes of visual impairment in neurofibromatosis are:
   - *Glaucoma* – uncommon and, when present, usually occurs at birth; it is frequently associated with an ipsilateral eyelid neurofibroma. Unless detected early it may cause blindness. Figure 12b shows advanced glaucomatous cupping of the optic disc.
   - *Glioma of the optic nerve* – typically presents between the ages of 4 and 8 years with a gradual onset of unilateral proptosis and visual loss.

   Note: other ocular features of neurofibromatosis are:
   - Bilateral melanocytic iris (Lisch) nodules – very common.
   - Choroidal naevi – in about one-third of patients.
   - Spheno-orbital encephalocele.
   - Plexiform neuroma of the orbit and eyelids.
   - Prominent corneal nerves.
   - Ectropion uveae.

Case 13

1. The signs are: vascularized red papules which have a butterfly distribution around the nose and cheeks. The diagnosis is *tuberous sclerosis* (epiloia or Bourneville's disease). The skin lesions (nodular fibroangiomas) are inconspicuous at birth but usually become clinically obvious between the ages of 2 and 5 years. On cursory examination they may be mistaken for acne vulgaris, hence the term 'adenoma sebaceum'.
2. Ocular lesions in patients with tuberous sclerosis are innocuous but may be helpful in establishing the diagnosis in very young children.
   - *Fundus astrocytomas* – in 50% of patients, involving both eyes in

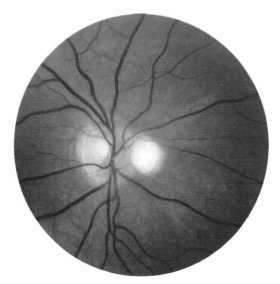

Figure 13b

15% of cases. They may be single or multiple and are most frequently situated near the optic disc (Figure 13b).
- *Hypopigmented iris spots* – common.
- *Hypopigmented fundus lesions* – uncommon.
3. Slowly growing *astrocytic hamartomas* of the central nervous system are a universal finding in patients with tuberous sclerosis. Although they may be found anywhere in the brain, they tend to concentrate in the periventricular area. Complications of hamartomas include:
- Epilepsy in 80%.
- Mental handicap in 60%.
- Hydrocephalus due to blockage of CSF circulation – uncommon.
- Malignant transformation – very rare.

Case 14

1. The signs are: patchy erythematous rash with vesicles and crusting involving the right forehead and side of the nose, and conjunctival hyperaemia. The diagnosis is *right herpes zoster ophthalmicus (HZO)*.
Note: Hutchinson's sign (involvement of the side of the nose in the distribution of the nasociliary branch of the ophthalmic division of the fifth nerve) is associated with an increased risk of eye complications.

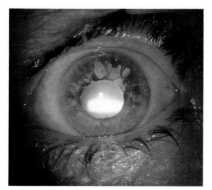

Figure 14b

2. About 50% of patients with HZO develop eye complications. A red eye may be caused by:
   - *Conjunctivitis* and *episcleritis* – both very common and innocuous.
   - *Scleritis* – uncommon but may become chronic.
   - *Keratitis* of various types – common. In some cases it may lead to diminished corneal sensation and the subsequent development of secondary corneal changes (neurotrophic keratitis).
   - *Iritis* – common; unless treated vigorously with topical steroids it may become chronic. Figure 14b shows iris atrophy due to HZO as seen against a red reflex.
3. *All cases of HZO must be referred to an ophthalmologist* because keratitis and iritis are difficult to diagnose with the naked eye and may require prolonged treatment.

Case 15

1. The signs are: bilateral erythematous maculopapular rash with crusting involving the face and lid margins, and redness and serous discharge of both eyes. The probable diagnosis is *Stevens–Johnson syndrome* (severe bullous erythema multiforme) which is characterized by:
   - Involvement of the oral mucosa – universal and characterized by bullae and erosions; on the lips these give rise to the characteristic haemorrhagic crusting.
   - Cutaneous involvement -- symmetrical erythematous maculopapules which may develop into target lesions.
   - Conjunctival involvement – 90% of cases.
2. In 50% of cases no precipitating factors are identified. In the remainder the most common aetiological agents are:
   - *Viruses.*

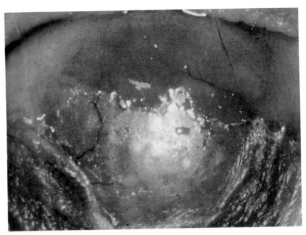

Figure 15b

- *Mycoplasma.*
- *Antibacterial agents* – particularly sulphonamides.
3. *The visual prognosis is variable.* The conjunctivitis in some patients may respond to intensive treatment with topical steroids. Other patients, however, subsequently develop focal red infarcts and yellow-white conjunctival membranes which on shedding leave focal fibrotic patches. Late rare complications are conjunctival fibrosis and keratinization, scarring of the eyelids, aberrant eyelashes and corneal scarring (Figure 15b).

Case 16

1. The signs are: conjunctival injection particularly in the lower fornix, discharge in the lower fornix, bright cornea and round pupil. The diagnosis is *conjunctivitis.*
2. The vast majority of patients with conjunctivitis have no associated systemic disease. The most common systemic associations are:
   - *Reiter's syndrome* – bilateral mucopurulent conjunctivitis which usually follows the urethritis but antedates the arthritis.
   - *Chlamydial infection* – follicular conjunctivitis which requires treatment with topical and systemic tetracycline.
   - *Cicatricial pemphigoid* – subacute conjunctivitis which becomes chronic.
   - *Stevens–Johnson syndrome* (see Case 15).
   - *Herpes zoster ophthalmicus* (see Case 14).
   - *Gonorrhoea* – very severe acute purulent conjunctivitis (Figure 16b).

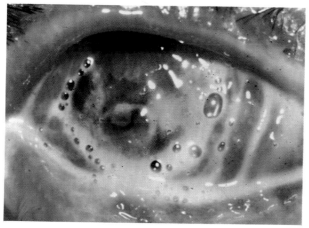

Figure 16b

3. *The visual prognosis varies* according to the underlying cause.
   - Simple bacterial conjunctivitis – innocuous; even without treatment it resolves within 10 days.
   - Reiter's syndrome conjunctivitis – transient and innocuous.
   - Chlamydial conjunctivitis – may be associated with keratitis.
   - Cicatricial pemphigoid – conjunctival scarring and shrinkage.
   - Stevens–Johnson syndrome (see Case 15).
   - Herpes zoster ophthalmicus (see Case 14).
   - Gonococcal conjunctivitis – may result in corneal perforation and blindness due to intraocular infection (endophthalmitis).

Case 17

1. The signs are: small punctate areas and larger mucous threads which have been stained with rose bengal dye. The dye is also taken up by the dry cells of the conjunctival epithelium. The diagnosis is *keratoconjunctivitis sicca* (KCS) in which there is deficient secretion of tears by the lacrimal glands.
   Note: the amount of secretion of tears can be measured by using a special strip of filter paper inserted inside the lower eyelids for 5 minutes (Schirmer's test – Figure 17b). Wetting of the filter paper of 10 mm or more is normal, 10–5 mm is suspicious and less than 5 mm is abnormal.
2. Patients with KCS can be divided into three main categories:
   - *Pure KCS* – only the eyes are involved.
   - *Primary Sjögren's syndrome* – an autoimmune disease characterized by the frequent presence of:

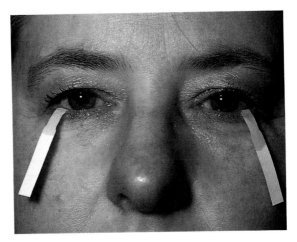

Figure 17b

- rheumatoid factor;
- antinuclear antibodies;
- hypergammaglobulinaemia;
- dry mouth (xerostomia);
- involvement of the bronchial and vaginal mucosa in some cases.
- *Secondary Sjögren's syndrome* – KCS is associated with one of the following systemic diseases:
  - rheumatoid arthritis;
  - systemic lupus erythematosus;
  - scleroderma;
  - sarcoidosis;
  - Crohn's disease.
3. Treatment of KCS is with the frequent instillation of *artificial tears* such as hypromellose. *Ointment* (Lacri-Lube) may also be helpful and, in very severe cases, *occlusion of the lacrimal puncta* may be required.

Case 18

1. The signs are: redness, a white fluid level in the bottom of the anterior chamber (hypopyon) and an irregular pupil due to an adhesion between the iris and the anterior surface of the lens (posterior synechiae).The diagnosis is *very severe acute anterior uveitis* (iritis). Photophobia is an early and characteristic symptom of acute iritis.
2. Many patients with acute iritis have no systemic association although they may carry HLA-B27. The main systemic associations are:
   - *Ankylosing spondylitis* (AS) – acute iritis affects about 30% of

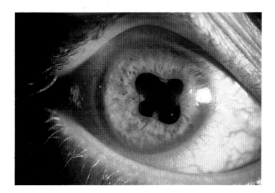

Figure 18b

patients with AS and conversely about 30% of patients with acute
iritis will have AS.
- *Reiter's syndrome* – acute iritis affects about 20% of patients.
- Behçet's disease – recurrent acute iritis with a transient hypopyon
  is common.
- *Sarcoidosis* – acute iritis typically affects young patients with
  acute sarcoid.
- *Secondary syphilis* – acute iritis affects about 5% of patients.
- *Ulcerative colitis* – an uncommon association.
- *Crohn's disease* – an uncommon association.

3. All patients with acute iritis must be referred immediately to an
   ophthalmologist for treatment with *steroid* and *mydriatic drops*.
   Figure 18b shows extensive posterior synechiae due to inappropriate treatment.

Case 19

1. The signs are: a white pupil (cataract), adhesions between the pupil
   and lens (posterior synechiae) and white corneal deposits (band
   keratopathy). The diagnosis is *chronic anterior uveitis with complications.*
2. Whilst some patients with chronic anterior uveitis are healthy, a
   significant percentage may have one of the following systemic
   disorders:
   - *Sarcoidosis* – chronic anterior uveitis more frequently than the
     acute type. The uveitis is characteristically granulomatous and
     frequently affects both eyes simultaneously. Chronic anterior
     uveitis usually occurs in older patients with chronic lung disease.
     Figure 19b shows iris nodules typical of granulomatous sarcoid
     anterior uveitis.
   - *Juvenile chronic arthritis* – by far the most common systemic
     association of chronic anterior uveitis in children. Patients who

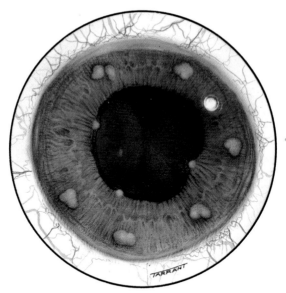

Figure 19b

are at increased risk of eye involvement are girls with a pauci-articular onset of arthritis who are also positive for circulating antinuclear antibodies.
- *Tuberculosis* – uncommon cause.
- *Syphilis* – uncommon cause.

3. Patients on long-term steroid drops should be monitored carefully by an ophthalmologist because of the possibility of the following complications:
- *Steroid-induced cataract.*
- *Steroid-induced glaucoma* which may occur in susceptible individuals.
- *Corneal complications* – bacterial, fungal and herpes simplex keratitis.

Case 20

1. The signs are: a large ulcer involving the inferior peripheral cornea. The diagnosis is *peripheral ulcerative keratitis.*
2. Severe peripheral ulcerative keratitis may occur as an isolated finding or it may be associated with:
- *Rheumatoid arthritis* – peripheral ulcerative keratitis is the second most common ocular complication affecting 2% of cases. The two main types are:
  - peripheral painless corneal guttering (contact lens cornea);

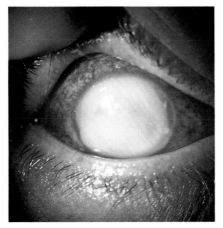

Figure 20b

– keratolysis characterized by painful, acute and severe ulceration.

- *Wegener's granulomatosis* – peripheral ulcerative keratitis is the most common ocular manifestation. Other ocular complications are: scleritis, conjunctivitis, orbital involvement, retinal vasculitis and anterior ischaemic optic neuropathy.
- *Polyarteritis nodosa* – a bilateral, progressive, necrotizing, peripheral, ulcerative keratitis may be the presenting feature. Other ocular complications are similar to Wegener's granulomatosis except for orbital involvement.
- *Systemic lupus erythematosus* – a rare association. Other ocular manifestations are: keratoconjunctivitis sicca, scleritis, retinal vasculitis and optic neuropathy.
3. Potential vision-threatening complications of corneal ulceration are:
- *Perforation of the cornea* – may lead to endophthalmitis (Figure 20b).
- *Severe corneal distortion* (astigmatism).

Case 21

1. The cornea shows deposits that appear in vortex fashion from a point below the pupil and swirl outwards. The diagnosis is *vortex keratopathy* (cornea verticillata)
2. The main causes of vortex keratopathy are drugs (chloroquine and amiodarone) and Fabry's disease. The patient may therefore have one of the following systemic disorders:
- *A rheumatological disorder* – treated with chloroquine.
- *A cardiac arrhythmia* – treated with amiodarone.
- *Fabry's disease* characterized by:

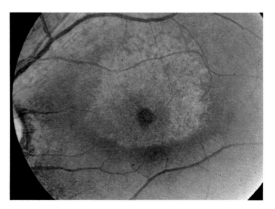

Figure 21b

  - angiokeratodermas;
  - cardiovascular and renal lesions;
  - episodes of excruciating pain involving the toes and fingers;
  - about 25% of patients have spoke-like lens opacities.
3. The presence of retinopathy *depends on the cause* of the corneal changes. If the patient has received long-term chloroquine therapy there is a small chance that he may also have chloroquine maculopathy. Figure 21b shows the typical bull's eye appearance in a patient with severe chloroquine retinotoxicity.
   Note:
   ● There is no correlation between chloroquine maculopathy and keratopathy.
   ● Chloroquine maculopathy is dose related – a cumulative dose of 100 g of chloroquine or a duration of treatment of less than 1 year is rarely associated with retinotoxicity.
   Neither amiodarone nor Fabry's disease is associated with retinopathy.

Case 22

1. The signs are: several areas of superior sclera thinning through which the underlying uveal tissue can be seen. The diagnosis is *scleromalacia perforans*. The condition starts with the formation of yellow necrotic patches in normal sclera until large areas of underlying uvea become exposed due to scleral thinning (Figure 22b).
   Note: other systemic diseases which may be associated with inflammatory scleritis, but not with scleromalacia perforans, are:
   ● Systemic lupus erythematosus.
   ● Wegener's granulomatosis.
   ● Polyarteritis nodosa.
   ● Herpes zoster ophthalmicus.

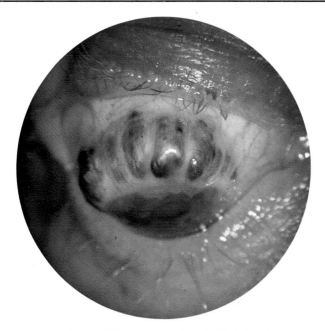

Figure 22b (Courtesy of Mr B. Mathalone)

2. The vast majority of patients with scleromalacia perforans are females with associated long-standing seropositive rheumatoid arthritis. Non-articular complications of rheumatoid arthritis include:
   - *Subcutaneous rheumatoid nodules.*
   - *Pleural effusions, interstitial lung fibrosis* and *lung nodules.*
   - *Felty's syndrome* (splenomegaly, leucopenia and thrombocytopenia).
   - *Acute pericarditis.*
   - *Vasculitis* of skin, peripheral nerves and viscera.
   - *Secondary amyloidosis.*
3. Patients with seropositive rheumatoid arthritis may also have:
   - Keratoconjunctivitis sicca (20%).
   - Keratitis (2%).

   Note: patients with rheumatoid arthritis are not at increased risk of developing anterior uveitis.

Case 23

1. The signs are: the lens is subluxated up and nasally but the zonules (suspensory lens ligaments) are intact. The most common systemic association is *Marfan's syndrome* in which lens subluxation is

present in about 70% of cases. The systemic features include:
- Mitral valve lesions and aortic aneurysms.
- Limbs disproportionately long as compared with trunk.
- High arched palate, arachnodactyly, hyperextensibility of joints, funnel or pigeon chest, flat feet and kyphoscoliosis.
- Muscular underdevelopment.
- Cystic lung lesions and recurrent pneumothorax.
- Small skin papules on the neck (Mieschler's elastomas).

2. Two other diseases which may be associated with lens subluxation are:
   - *Homocystinuria* – lens subluxation is common and is usually downward with complete disintegration of the zonules. Systemic features include:
     - increased platelet stickiness;
     - arachnodactyly and osteoporosis;
     - mental handicap;
     - malar flush and fine hair.
   - *Ehlers–Danlos syndrome* – lens subluxation is uncommon. Systemic features include:
     - bleeding diathesis;
     - dissecting aneurysm and mitral valve prolapse;
     - hyperextensibility of joints, flat feet, kyphoscoliosis and genu recurvatum;
     - thin and hyperextensible skin;
     - diaphragmatic hernias;
     - diverticula of gastrointestinal and respiratory tracts.

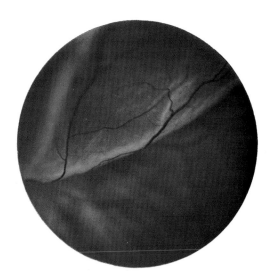

Figure 23b

3. Other ocular complications of Marfan's syndrome are:
   - *Glaucoma.*
   - *Hypoplasia of the dilator pupillae.*
   - *Myopia.*
   - *Retinal detachment* (Figure 23b).

Case 24

1. The diagnosis is *cataract.*
2. Systemic associations:
   - *Diabetes mellitus* is associated with two types of cataracts:
     - accelerated senile cataract in which the patient develops lens opacities at a younger age than in a non-diabetic patient;
     - true diabetic cataract (very rare) in which the entire lens may become completely opaque (mature) within a few days.

   Note: occasionally unstable diabetics develop frequent changes in refraction. Hyperglycaemia may cause myopia in which the patient suddenly develops blurring of distance vision but is able to read without reading spectacles.
   - *Systemic steroids* – if used long term.
   - *Dystrophia myotonica* – frequently associated with presenile posterior subcapsular stellate (Christmas-tree cataracts).
   - *Atopic dermatitis* – occasionally associated.
   - *Miscellaneous*:
     - Down's syndrome;

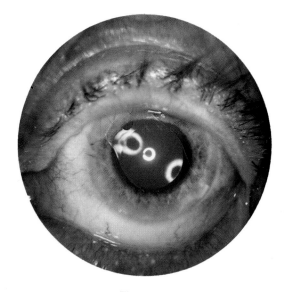

Figure 24b

- galactosaemia and galactokinase deficiency;
- Fabry's disease;
- Wilson's disease;
- hypocalcaemia;
- maternal infections (rubella, toxoplasmosis and cytomegalo-virus) may cause infantile cataracts.

3. Treatment is by *cataract extraction* and the implantation of an artificial lens (implant). Figure 24b shows the appearance of an eye with an implant.

Case 25

1. The signs are: a normal optic disc – pink colour, small round central cup, well-defined margins and clear visibility of the superficial disc blood vessels and peripapillary retinal nerve fibre striations. The most probable diagnosis is *retrobulbar neuritis.*
   Note: the prognosis is excellent in the vast majority of cases with a return to normal or near normal vision within 6–8 weeks. Treatment is usually unecessary although steroids speed up the rate of visual recovery.

2. Between 50% and 70% of patients with isolated optic neuritis will have an abnormal MRI similar to that seen in *multiple sclerosis* (MS). Seventy-four per cent of women and 34% of men with optic neuritis will develop MS when followed up for 15 years. Other risk factors for subsequent MS are:
   - Winter onset.
   - Presence of HLA-DR2.
   - Uhthoff's phenomenon (worsening of visual acuity when body temperature rises or during physical exercise).

3. Potential subsequent ocular complications of MS are:
   - *Internuclear ophthalmoplegia* characterized by:
     - defective adduction of the ipsilateral eye;

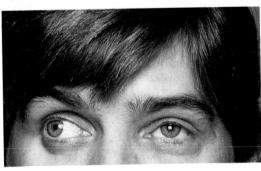

Figure 25b (Courtesy of Mr P. Rosen)

– ataxic nystagmus of the contralateral eye;
– usually normal convergence.

Figure 25b shows a patient with a left internuclear ophthalmo-plegia.

- *Isolated ocular motor nerve palsies.*
- *Nystagmus.*
- *Conjugate gaze palsies.*

Case 26

1. The diagnosis is severe *optic atrophy.*
2. The history of slowly progressive visual failure is suggestive of a compressive lesion of either the ipsilateral optic nerve or chiasm or both. The most common lesions are:
   - *Meningiomas* – typically affect middle-aged women; those arising from the optic nerve sheath, olfactory groove or the sphen-oidal ridge will preferentially damage the optic nerve, whilst those arising from the tuberculum sellae may compress either the optic nerve or chiasm.
   - *Pituitary tumours, craniopharyngiomas* and *aneurysms* – also frequent causes of chiasmal or optic nerve compression.
3. Investigations include:
   - *Visual field examination:*
     - an upper temporal defect in the left eye would suggest a lesion at the junction of the chiasm and optic nerve of the right eye (junctional scotoma);
     - a bilateral hemianopic temporal visual field defect which is denser above would be indicative of chiasmal compression from below (Figure 26b).

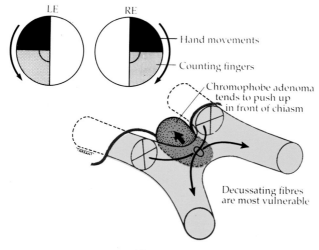

Figure 26b

– a bilateral hemianopic temporal visual field defect which is denser below would suggest a craniopharyngioma.
- *CT* and *MRI* of the optic nerve and parachiasmal region.
- *Endocrinological evaluation* – tailored to the individual patient.

Case 27

1. The signs are: the optic disc is hyperaemic, it has a small cup, its margins are indistinct particularly nasally, and a small peripapillary flame-shaped haemorrhage is present inferiorly. The diagnosis is *papilloedema.*
   Note: papilloedema is defined as disc swelling secondary to raised intracranial pressure. It is nearly always bilateral, although it may be asymmetrical. All other causes of disc oedema not associated with raised intracranial pressure are referred to as 'disc swelling'.
2. The main causes of papilloedema are:
   - *Intracranial mass* – should be suspected in all patients until the contrary is proved. Tumours of the cerebral hemispheres tend to produce papilloedema later than those in the posterior fossa.
   - *Benign intracranial hypertension* (pseudotumour cerebri).
   - *Miscellaneous*:
     – encephalopathy due to lead poisoning;
     – carbon dioxide retention in chronic lung disease;
     – hypoparathyroidism;
     – Guillain–Barré syndrome.

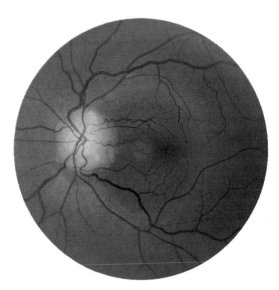

Figure 27b

3. The main condition which may be mistaken for early papilloedema is *optic disc drusen* (Figure 27b) which is characterized by:
   - Anomalous branching of the blood vessels emerging from the disc.
   - Absence of obscuration of small blood vessels crossing the disc.
   - Absent optic cup.
   - Pink or yellow colour of the optic disc.
   - 'Lumpy' appearance at the margins of the disc.

Case 28

1. The signs are: the optic disc is pale and swollen and there is a small flame-shaped haemorrhage at the disc margin at 11 o'clock. The diagnosis is *anterior ischaemic optic neuropathy* (AION) which may be of either an arteritic or a non-arteritic type.
   Note: the pale appearance of the optic disc should not be confused with that due to opaque (myelinated) nerve fibres (Figure 28b).
2. Even in the absence of other symptoms suggestive of giant cell arteritis (e.g. jaw claudication, polymyalgia rheumatica), it is extremely important to exclude this diagnosis because occasionally the condition presents with blindness and, unless treated, there is a high risk of bilateral involvement.
   Special investigations include:
   - *Blood tests*: ESR, C-reactive protein, Hb, WBC, alkaline phosphatase and antinuclear antibodies.

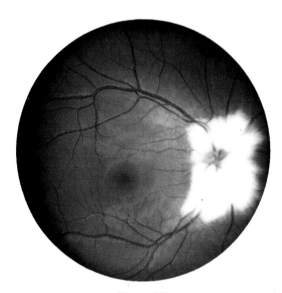

Figure 28b

- *Temporal artery biopsy* – for histological confirmation.
3. *Treatment depends on the cause.*
  - Non-arteritic AION – does *not benefit* from any form of treatment.
  - Arteritic AION – treated with *systemic steroids* as follows:
    - immediate intravenous hydrocortisone 250 mg and oral pred-nisolone 80 mg for 3 days;
    - then 60 mg for 3 days and 40 mg for 4 days;
    - subsequently the daily dose is reduced by 5 mg weekly until 10 mg is reached;
    - maintenance daily therapy is 10 mg initially for 12 months;
    - subsequent therapy is determined by patient's symptoms and ESR.

Case 29

1. The signs are: the fundus shows several minute golden lesions consisting of cholesterol crystals in the lumen of an arteriole. The diagnosis is very suggestive of retinal ischaemia due to *recurrent embolization* (amaurosis fugax). The main types of retinal emboli are:
   - Cholesterol crystals (Hollenhorst's plaques) – indicative of atheromatous disease in the great vessels (usually asympto-matic).
   - White emboli composed of platelets and fibrin – usually the cause of amaurosis fugax. They are seldom seen in the retina, although occasionally they may give rise to transient cotton-wool spots.

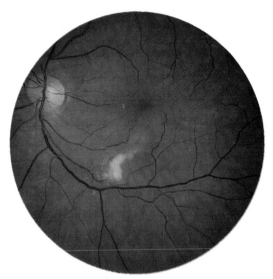

Figure 29b

Figure 29b shows a cotton-wool spot associated with an embolic occlusion of the left inferotemporal artery.
- Calcific emboli which usually arise from either a calcified aortic valve or the ascending aorta – may cause a major arterial obstruction.
- Miscellaneous emboli in association with mural thrombi, mitral leaflet prolapse, atrial myxoma and vegetations.

2. The presence of amaurosis fugax in a patient of this age group is very suggestive of atheromatous ulceration and stenosis at the bifurcation of the common carotid artery in the neck. Patients with retinal TIAs may also develop *cerebral TIAs* and about 15% of patients with cerebral TIAs develop *stroke, myocardial infarction* or *death* within 2 years.

3. Investigations of patients with amaurosis fugax include:
- *Blood pressure.*
- *Urinalysis.*
- *Palpation* and *auscultation* of the *arteries in the neck.*
- *Special investigations* include:
  - duplex scanning;
  - digital intravenous subtraction angiography;
  - magnetic resonance vascular imaging;
  - arterial angiography.

Case 30

1. The signs are: generalized pallor of the fundus except at the macula and extreme attenuation of the retinal arterioles. The inferotemporal branch is white and completely devoid of blood. The diagnosis is *acute central retinal artery occlusion.*

2. This is a medical emergency which should be treated as follows:
- *Lie the patient flat* to help maintain the circulation to the eye.
- *Apply firm ocular massage* intermittently every 10 seconds for at least 15 minutes to lower the intraocular pressure and thereby increase blood flow and also dislodge emboli (if present).
- *Give an intravenous injection of acetazolamide* (Diamox) 500 mg to further lower the intraocular pressure.

  Unfortunately despite these measures the visual prognosis is very poor.

3. The possible underlying systemic causes are:
- *Atherosclerosis of the central retinal artery* – by far the most common.
- *Embolization* – usually by calcific emboli arising from either calcified aortic heart valves or from the ascending aorta.
- *Arteritis* – giant cell arteritis, systemic lupus erythematosus, polyarteritis nodosa and Wegener's granulomatosis may cause retinal artery occlusion as well as anterior ischaemic optic

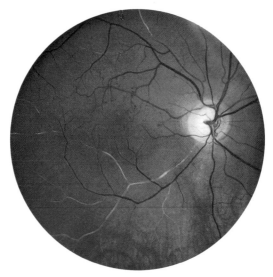

Figure 30b

neuropathy. Figure 30b shows an old complete arterial occlusion of the inferotemporal branch and a terminal occlusion of the supero-temporal branch in a 43-year-old man with polyarteritis nodosa.

Case 31

1. The signs are: attenuation of the superotemporal retinal artery and a few small flame-shaped haemorrhages near the disc. The diagnosis is *hypertensive retinopathy*.
2. The primary response of the retinal arterioles in hypertension is narrowing. However, the degree of narrowing is dependent on the extent of pre-existing replacement fibrosis (involutional sclerosis). For this reason, hypertensive narrowing in its purest form is seen only in young individuals. In sustained severe hypertension the following lesions may be seen:
   - *Cotton-wool spots* – due to obstruction of precapillary arterioles.
   - *Vascular leakage* – flame-shaped haemorrhages, retinal oedema and hard exudates; the radial deposition of hard ex-udates in the fovea in Henle's layer may lead to the formation of a macular star.
   - *Disc swelling* – the hallmark of malignant hypertension.
   - *Arteriosclerotic changes* – due to thickening of the vessel wall. Figure 31b shows malignant hypertension in the right fundus of a 35-year-old woman. There is disc swelling, retinal oedema involving the nasal retina, hard exudation at the macula and constriction of the arterioles.

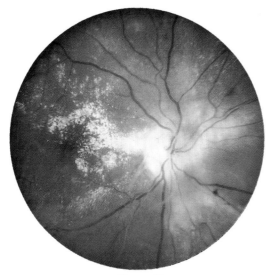

Figure 31b

3. Other ocular complications in hypertensive patients are:
   - *Retinal vein occlusion.*
   - *Retinal artery macroaneurysm.*
   - *Non-arteritic anterior ischaemic optic neuropathy.*
   - *Ocular motor nerve palsies.*
   - *Worsening of diabetic retinopathy.*

Case 32

1. The signs are: swelling of the optic disc, many scattered flame-shaped haemorrhages, cotton-wool spots and venous dilatation. The diagnosis is *central retinal vein occlusion.*
2. Whilst many patients with retinal vein occlusion have no associated systemic disease, the condition may be associated with the following:
   - *Hypertension* – this is associated with an increased risk of both branch retinal vein occlusion and central retinal vein occlusion. It has been postulated that the vein is compressed by the thickened artery where the two share a common adventitia (i.e. just behind the lamina cribrosa of the optic disc and at arteriovenous crossing in the fundus). Figure 32b shows a left branch retinal vein occlusion with flame-shaped haemorrhages and a cotton-wool spot at the posterior pole.
   - *Blood dyscrasias* – associated with either hypercellularity (chronic leukaemia, polycythaemia) or changes in plasma

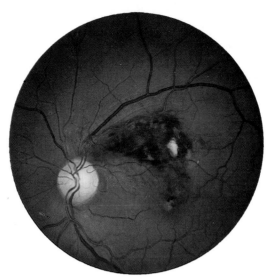

Figure 32b

proteins (Waldenström's macroglobulinaemia) may rarely precipitate retinal vein occlusion.
- *Vasculitis* of the retinal veins (periphlebitis) – in sarcoidosis and Behçet's disease may, if severe, occlude the retinal veins.
- *Sickle-cell disease* – occasional cause.
3. *The visual prognosis is poor* in a central retinal vein occlusion due to associated retinal ischaemia. Some patients also develop an intractable type of (neovascular) glaucoma in which new blood vessels grow on the surface of the iris and cause the intraocular pressure to rise by impairing the outflow of aqueous humour from the eye. Neovascular glaucoma does not occur following a branch vein occlusion.

Case 33

1. The signs are: fundus shows many small yellowish dots at the posterior pole. The diagnosis is *colloid bodies* (drusen) of the macula. Colloid bodies are rare in patients under the age of 45 years, uncommon between the ages of 45 and 60 and fairly common thereafter.
2. *Referral to an ophthalmologist is unnecessary* in patients with colloid bodies and normal vision because no treatment is required. On cursory examination, colloid bodies may be mistaken for hard exudates due to background diabetic retinopathy by the inexperienced observer.

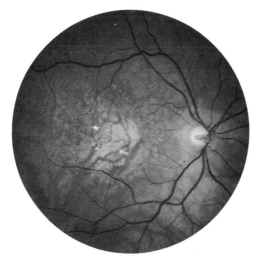

Figure 33b

3. In the vast majority of patients, the *long-term visual prognosis is excellent* and only a small minority develop further degenerative changes at the macula (senile or age-related macular degeneration) which cause impairment of central vision. Figure 33b shows atrophic changes at the macula in a patient with macular degeneration.

Case 34

1. The signs are: the fundus shows a few hard exudates, microaneurysms and haemorrhages temporal to the fovea. The diagnosis is *mild background diabetic retinopathy*. This is by far the most common type and is caused by microvascular leakage into the retina. In the absence of maculopathy it is asymptomatic.
2. *Referral to an ophthalmologist is unnecessary* because visual acuity is normal and the lesions are not threatening the fovea. The patient should have an annual fundus examination and measurement of visual acuity.
3. The earliest features of background diabetic retinopathy are *microaneurysms* which appear as small, round, red dots, usually located temporal to the macula. They vary in size from 20 to 200 μm in diameter. Large microaneurysms may be difficult to distinguish from dot haemorrhages.

    Other features of background DR are:
    - Dot and blot haemorrhages located within the compact deep retinal layers.
    - Hard exudates – more advanced lesions which are frequently

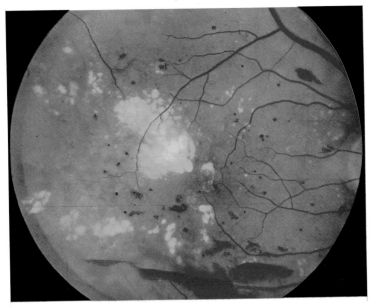

Figure 34b

located in a circinate pattern peripheral to areas of chronic intraretinal leakage from microaneurysms.

- Diffuse retinal oedema which causes a diffuse thickening of the retina; this is difficult to detect, particularly by the non-expert.

Figure 34b shows a composite picture of the various lesions of background diabetic retinopathy. A flame-shaped haemorrhage above the disc and preretinal haemorrhages inferiorly are also present.

Case 35

1. The diagnosis is background diabetic retinopathy with involvement of the macula by hard exudates (*diabetic maculopathy*). Maculopathy is the most common cause of visual impairment in patients with diabetic retinopathy and is more frequent in NIDDs than in IDDs. It results from involvement of the fovea by oedema and/or hard exudates. The symptoms are a gradual impairment of central vision such as difficulty in reading small print or seeing road signs.

2. All patients with diabetes who have impaired vision which cannot be improved by the provision of spectacles *should be referred to an ophthalmologist* (non-urgent) because laser photocoagulation

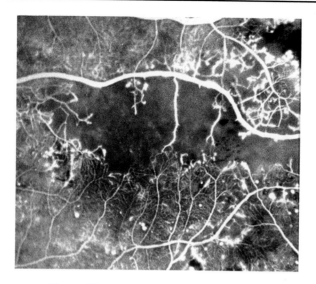

Figure 35b (Courtesy of Mr R. Whitelocke)

will stabilize (but seldom improve) visual acuity in about 50% of cases.

3. The ophthalmologist may wish to perform *fluorescein angiography* in selected patients. In this procedure fluorescein is injected into a vein and then photographs are taken as the dye passes through the retinal circulation. Fluorescein angiography is helpful in determining the site and extent of leakage into the macula as well as the presence and severity of macular ischaemia. If there is significant retinal ischaemia at the macula then photocoagulation is contraindicated. Figure 35b shows a fluorescein angiogram of severe ischaemic maculopathy.

Case 36

1. The fundus shows *severe background diabetic retinopathy*. The main retinal veins are slightly dilated and there is one cotton-wool spot at the bifurcation of the inferotemporal vein. The latter two signs are indicative of moderately severe retinal hypoxia characteristic of pre-proliferative diabetic retinopathy.

2. Although laser treatment is usually unnecessary the *patient should be referred to an ophthalmologist* (non-urgent) because a close follow-up is required so that proliferative changes can be detected and treated early. Figure 36b shows a composite picture of the clinical features of pre-proliferative diabetic retinopathy. It is important to emphasize that not all features will necessarily be present in the same patient.

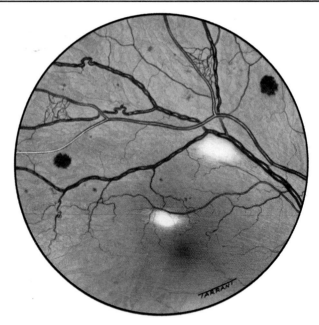

Figure 36b

- Cotton-wool spots due to capillary closure in the retinal nerve fibre layer.
- Intraretinal microvascular abnormalities.
- Venous changes – dilatation, beading, looping and sausage-like segmentation.
- Arteriolar narrowing which may resemble branch retinal vein occlusion.
- Large, dark, blot haemorrhages due to haemorrhagic retinal infarcts.

3. Diabetic retinopathy may be worsened by:
   - *Pregnancy.*
   - *Poorly controlled hypertension.*
   - *Renal disease.*
   - *Anaemia.*

Case 37

1. The fundus shows moderate flat new vessels at the optic disc indicative of *proliferative diabetic retinopathy*. This is less common but potentially more serious than the background type and typically affects IDDs. Proliferative diabetic retinopathy is associated with severe retinal hypoxia and is asymptomatic in the absence of complications (i.e. vitreous haemorrhage and retinal detachment).

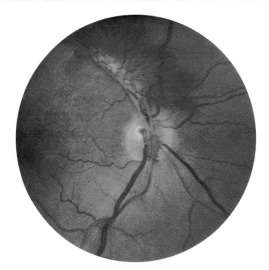

Figure 37b

Initially the new vessels are bare and flat and easy to miss on cursory examination. Later they may become elevated and may be associated with a fibrous component which is easier to detect. Figure 37b shows severe fibrovascular proliferation extending from the optic disc along the superotemporal arcade.

2. *Referral to an ophthalmologist is necessary* (urgent) because the patient will require laser therapy to prevent complications.
3. Other ocular complications in diabetic patients are:
   - *Cataracts* – accelerated senile or true diabetic (see Case 24).
   - *Isolated ocular motor nerve palsies* – frequently caused by diabetes; a pupil-sparing third nerve palsy, which may be painful (see Case 2), is common, as is a sixth nerve palsy (see Case 4).
   - *Pupillary abnormalities* – in IDDs due to an autonomic neuro-pathy of the pupil; characteristically the reaction to near is better than that to light (light–near dissociation).
   - *Frequent changes in refraction* – a feature of unstable diabetes.
   - *Neovascularization of the iris* (rubeosis iridis).

Case 38

1. Laser photocoagulation is essentially a destructive form of therapy in which *light energy is absorbed by ocular pigments and con-verted into heat energy*. Photocoagulation is performed at a slit lamp and the light is focused onto the retina by a special lens held by the ophthalmologist.
2. The two main indications for laser therapy are:
   - *Maculopathy* – provided it is not too advanced and not associated

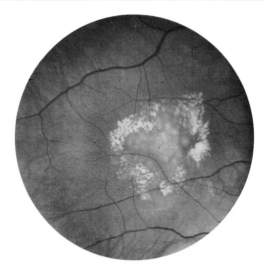

Figure 38b

with severe macular ischaemia. Maculopathy is treated by focal burns to areas of leakage. The results are reasonably good with stabilization of visual acuity in about 50% of cases. Improvement of vision is, however, rare. Figure 38b shows several recently applied laser burns to leaking microaneurysms located inside a ring of hard exudates.

- *Proliferative diabetic retinopathy* – this is usually progressive unless treated by photocoagulation. Treatment is by panretinal photocoagulation in which several hundred burns are applied to large areas of the peripheral retina. The results are good provided the condition is not too advanced and involution of neovascularization is achieved in up to 80% of patients.

3. Potential complications of laser therapy are:
- *Macular damage* – oedema, pucker or accidental burns.
- *Retinal detachment* – due to contraction of fibrous tissue.
- *Effects on visual function* – night blindness, constriction of visual fields, alteration of colour vision and diminished light brightness appreciation.

Case 39

1. The signs are: visualization of the temporal and inferior fundus obscured by vitreous haemorrhage; the optic disc shows severe neovascularization and old laser scars are evident outside the temporal vascular arcades. The diagnosis is *vitreous haemorrhage from disc new vessels* which have not regressed despite laser therapy.

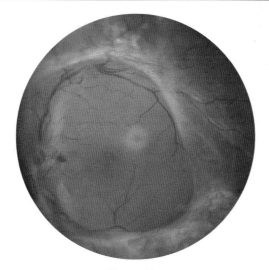

Figure 39b

2. Management is as follows:
   - The patient should be asked to *rest* in order to enhance the speed of absorption of the vitreous haemorrhage.
   - Once the haemorrhage has absorbed, *further laser photocoagulation* will be required in order to cause involution of the new vessels.
   - If the vitreous haemorrhage does not absorb after several months, or if it increases in density, then excision of the blood from the eye can be considered (*pars plana vitrectomy*).
3. The three main causes of severe and persistent visual impairment in diabetic patients are:
   - *Tractional retinal detachment* – caused by contraction of fibrovascular tissue. Treatment is by pars plana vitrectomy. Figure 39b shows an extensive tractional retinal detachment in a patient with proliferative diabetic retinopathy.
   - *Severe vitreous haemorrhage.*
   - *Neovascular glaucoma* (see Case 32).

Case 40

1. The signs are: fluffy white exudate surrounding the veins and retinal haemorrhages. The diagnosis is *retinal vasculitis*. Vasculitis may involve the retinal vein (periphlebitis) or, less commonly, the retinal arterioles (arteritis).
2. Retinal periphlebitis may be associated with the following:
   - *Sarcoidosis* – typically involves the retinal veins and, in severe cases, the perivascular accumulation of granulomatous tissue

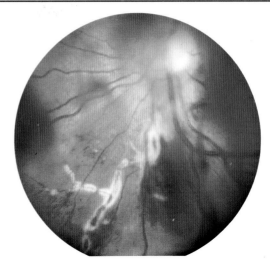

Figure 40b (Courtesy of Mr J. Shilling)

may give rise to 'candlewax drippings' or 'candlewax exudates'. Figure 40b shows 'candlewax exudates' and vitreous
haemorrhage in a patient with sarcoidosis.
- *Behçet's disease* – may be associated with periphlebitis which
  may lead to occlusion of major vessels.
- *Tuberculosis* – a rare cause.
3. Other ocular complications will *depend on the cause of the vasculitis.*
   - Sarcoidosis – eyelid plaques (lupus pernio), conjunctival granu-
     lomata, lacrimal gland involvement, anterior uveitis (acute or
     chronic), choroidal and optic nerve granulomata.
   - Behçet's – anterior uveitis and retinitis.
   - Tuberculosis – chronic granulomatous anterior uveitis and chor-
     oidal granulomata.

Case 41

1. The signs are: a yellowish lesion with ill-defined borders is present
   just above the macula and an area of pigmentation along the
   superotemporal arcade. The diagnosis is *active posterior uveitis*
   (retinochoroiditis).
2. The most common cause of posterior uveitis in the UK is *reactivation
   of congenital toxoplasmosis.* The active lesion usually heals within
   1–4 months (except in AIDS patients) and leaves an atrophic scar
   surrounded by pigment (Figure 41b).
   Note: treatment of vision-threatening lesions located near the

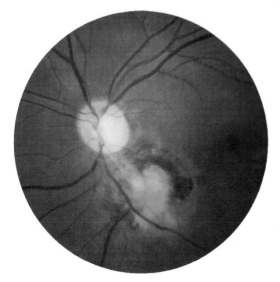

Figure 41b

macula or optic nerve is with a combination of pyrimethamine, clindamycin and sulphonamides. In certain very severe cases systemic steroids are also used.
3. Other systemic diseases associated with posterior uveitis are:
   - *Behçet's disease* – may cause a transient retinitis as well as a periphlebitis.
   - *Sarcoidosis and tuberculosis* – choroidal granulomata.
   - *AIDS* – cytomegalovirus retinitis.
   - *Syphilis* – rare cause.
   - *Candidiasis* – particularly in intravenous drug abusers.
   - *Whipple's disease* – very rare cause.

Case 42

1. The signs are: area of retinitis and haemorrhage involving the superior fundus. The most probable diagnosis is *cytomegalovirus (CMV) retinitis*.
2. The most common systemic association of CMV retinitis is *AIDS*. CMV retinitis occurs in about 45% of AIDS patients and is frequently bilateral. Its appearance is a grave prognostic sign as most patients are dead within a few months of its development.
   The clinical appearance of CMV retinitis is variable:
   - Cotton-wool spots – frequently the initial lesions.
   - Central retinitis – dense, white, well-demarcated area of retinal necrosis which frequently develops along the vascular arcades

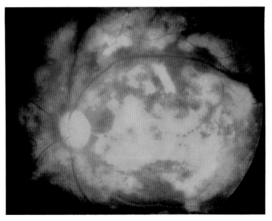

Figure 42b (Courtesy of Mr R. Marsh)

and may contain flame-shaped haemorrhages – as in this patient.
- Peripheral retinitis – more granular and less intense.

Note: irrespective of whether the retinitis starts centrally or in the periphery it spreads slowly but relentlessly until the entire fundus is completely involved (Figure 42b).

3. CMV retinitis is initially treated with *intravenous ganciclovir*. Unfortunately recurrences are very common following cessation of treatment. In very severe cases intravitreal injections may be tried.

Case 43

1. The signs are: linear streaks with serrated edges that are darker than the retinal blood vessels. The diagnosis is *angioid streaks* which are associated with breaks in the thin (Bruch's) membrane that separates the retinal pigment epithelium from the underlying choroid.
2. Patients with angioid streaks may lose vision in one of three ways:
   - *Subretinal haemorrhage* due to rupture of a subretinal blood vessel at the macula (Figure 43b). These blood vessels are derived from the choroidal circulation. They pass through the defect in Bruch's membrane associated with the angioid streak and grow under the retina.
   - *Macular involvement by a streak*.
   - *Macular haemorrhage* – due to a traumatic choroidal rupture.
3. About 50% of patients with angioid streaks have no systemic association. In order of frequency the remainder may have one of the following conditions:

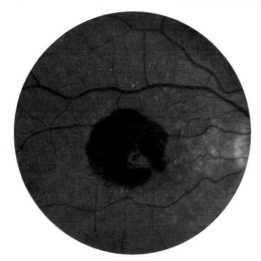

Figure 43b

- *Pseudoxanthoma elasticum* – by far the most common association (Gröndblad–Strandberg syndrome). The main systemic features are:
  - skin lesions consisting of small yellow papules;
  - cardiovascular disease due to accelerated atherosclerosis;
  - haemorrhage from the gastrointestinal and urinary tracts.
- *Paget's disease* – angioid streaks in about 10% of cases.
- *Ehlers–Danlos syndrome* (see Case 23).
- *Sickle-cell disease.*

Case 44

1. The signs are: clumps of retinal pigment which have a bone-corpuscle shape and attenuation of the arterioles. The diagnosis is *retinitis pigmentosa.*
2. The two main symptoms of retinitis pigmentosa are:
   - *Night blindness* – difficulty in adapting to dim illumination such as when entering a dark room.
   - *Difficulties with side vision* – due to constriction of both visual fields.

   Note: patients with retinitis pigmentosa may also have visual impairment due to:
   - cataract;
   - glaucoma;
   - maculopathy;
   - conical cornea (keratoconus).

   Figure 44b shows bulging of the left lower eyelid due to keratoconus (Munson's sign).

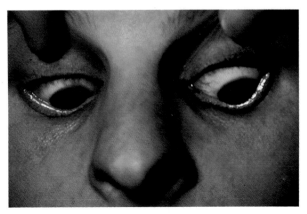

Figure 44b

3. Systemic associations of retinitis pigmentosa include:
   - *Bassen–Kornzweig syndrome* – abetalipoproteinaemia, fat malabsorption, spinocerebellar ataxia and acanthocytosis.
   - *Refsum's syndrome* – hypertrophic peripheral neuropathy, cerebellar ataxia, CSF cytoalbuminous inversion, deafness and ichthyosis.
   - *Laurence–Moon–Biedl syndrome* – mental handicap, obesity, hypogonadism, polydactyly and syndactyly.
   - *Friedreich's ataxia* – posterior column disease, ataxia and nystagmus.
   - *Kearns–Sayre syndrome* – ocular myopathy and heart block.
   - *Usher's syndrome* – congenital non-progressive sensorineural deafness.

Case 45

1. The signs are: two very tortuous and dilated retinal blood vessels leading to a peripheral lesion. These findings occur in *retinal capillary haemangioma*. About 25% of patients with retinal haemangiomas have associated systemic lesions (*von Hippel–Lindau syndrome*).
2. Although retinal haemangiomas are benign they grow and leak and without treatment they may cause the following vision-threatening complications:
   - *Deposition of hard exudate at the macula.*
   - *Vitreous haemorrhage.*
   - *Exudative retinal detachment.*

   Figure 45b shows shrinking of the retinal blood vessels following treatment of the tumour by laser photocoagulation.

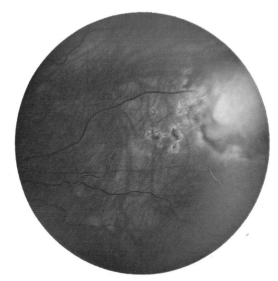

Figure 45b

3. The von Hippel–Lindau syndrome is dominantly inherited. The patient's brother may be ataxic because of *haemangioblastoma* which may involve the cerebellum, medulla, pons or spinal cord.

Other systemic complications in patients with the von Hippel-Lindau syndrome include:
- Cysts of the kidneys, pancreas, liver, epididymis, ovary and lung.
- Hypernephroma.
- Phaeochromocytoma.
- Polycythaemia.

Case 46

1. The signs are: an oval, slightly elevated, creamy-white, subretinal lesion with ill-defined borders. The diagnosis is a *metastatic carcinoma to the choroid*.

Note:
- The breast is the most common primary site in females and the bronchus in males.
- A choroidal secondary may be the initial presentation of a bronchial carcinoma but a past history of mastectomy is the rule in patients with breast tumours.
- Other less common primary sites are the kidney, testis and gastrointestinal tract.
- The prostate is an extremely rare primary site.

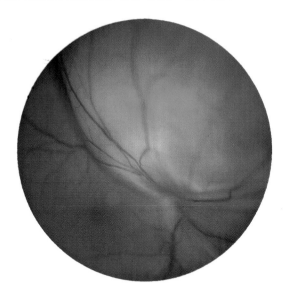

Figure 46b

2. Choroidal metastases should be differentiated from primary amelanotic melanomas of the choroid. In contrast to metastases these are invariably unilateral. Figure 46b shows a primary amelanotic choroidal melanoma.
3. Other ocular manifestations of metastatic carcinoma are:
   - *Hemianopia* – CNS metastases.
   - *Horner's syndrome* – Pancoast's tumour (see Case 2).
   - *Diplopia* – ocular motor nerve involvement.
   - *Ptosis* – Eaton–Lambert syndrome.
   - *Carcinomatous optic neuropathy* – very rare.

Case 47

1. The signs are: one round black subretinal lesion and several smaller clumps of pigment. The diagnosis is *congenital hypertrophy of the retinal pigment epithelium.*
2. There is an association between *familial polyposis coli* and congenital hypertrophy of the retinal pigment epithelium. Familial polyposis coli is a dominantly inherited condition characterized by multiple adenomatous polyps of the colon. Virtually all patients with this condition develop carcinoma of the colon by the age of 50 years. Because of the dominant inheritance pattern, an intensive survey of family members must be conducted. The presence of retinal lesions in family members should arouse suspicion of polyposis coli.

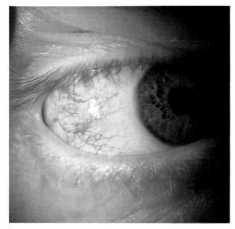

Figure 47b

3. Ocular complications in bowel disorders include:
   - *Ulcerative colitis* – acute anterior uveitis; the incidence of uveitis is increased when ulcerative colitis and ankylosing spondylitis coexist in the same patient.
   - *Crohn's disease* – anterior uveitis and episcleritis.
   Figure 47b shows a localized area of dilated blood vessels characteristic of simple episcleritis.
   - *Whipple's disease* – chronic anterior uveitis, vitritis and posterior uveitis.

Case 48

1. The fundus shows *clumps of hyperpigmentation*.
2. These changes are characteristic of *thioridazine* (Melleril) retinotoxicity. This drug may be toxic to the retina when a daily dose of 800 mg is exceeded, but retinotoxicity is unrelated to the total cumulative dose.
3. Other potentially toxic drugs are:
   - *Chloroquine* (see Case 21).
   - *Tamoxifen* – used in the treatment of breast carcinoma. Retinotoxicity in the form of multiple paramacular refractive lesions may develop in some patients. The retinal lesions, if severe, may cause visual impairment. Bilateral optic neuritis, which is reversible on cessation, is also a rare complication. Figure 48b shows advanced tamoxifen retinopathy.
   - *Ethambutol* – used in the treatment of tuberculosis. About 1% of patients develop optic neuropathy on a dose of 15 mg/kg per day. The risk is increased with higher doses, particularly if the

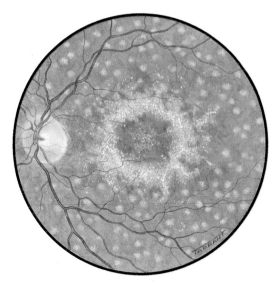

Figure 48b

patient has associated renal failure. Patients with optic neuropathy may have normal discs or they may show disc oedema and splinter-shaped haemorrhages.

- *Chlorpromazine* – only if extremely high doses of over 2400 mg/day are taken over a long period of time.

Case 49

1. The blood film shows an acute *lymphocytic leukaemia.*
2. The main causes of a red eye in patients with acute lymphocytic leukaemia are:

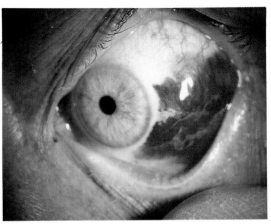

Figure 49b

- *Spontaneous subconjunctival haemorrhage* – associated with low blood platelets (Figure 49b).
- *Spontaneous haemorrhage into the anterior chamber of the eye* (hyphaemia).
- *Iritis* – may be associated with hypopyon.
3. Other ocular complications of acute leukaemia are:
- *Orbital infiltration* – in acute and chronic leukaemias (more common in the former particularly if lymphocytic).
- *Retinopathy* – venous dilatation and tortuosity, flame-shaped haemorrhages, Roth's spots and cotton-wool spots; the latter may be due either to leukaemic infiltration of the retina or to associated anaemia.
- *Optic neuropathy* – fluffy infiltration of the optic disc with variable oedema and haemorrhage.

Case 50

1. The blood film shows a *megaloblastic anaemia*.
2. Patients with megaloblastic anaemias may develop visual failure due to *optic neuropathy* which is characterized by bilateral centrocaecal scotoma (i.e. extending around the blind spot and fixation).
3. Megaloblastic anaemias, as well as anaemias of other types, may give rise to *retinopathy* which is usually innocuous and rarely of diagnostic importance. The clinical features include:
- Flame-shaped haemorrhages.
- Cotton-wool spots.
- Roth's spots.

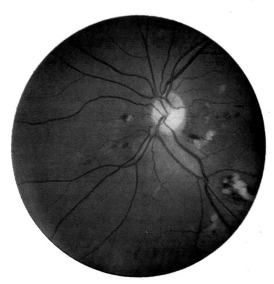

Figure 50b

- Venous tortuosity which seems to be directly related to the level of the haematocrit or the severity of anaemia.

Figure 50b shows flame-shaped haemorrhages, cotton-wool spots and slight tortuosity of the inferotemporal vein in the left eye of a patient with severe anaemia.

Index

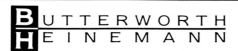